THE GIFT OF A CHILD

A GUIDE TO DONOR INSEMINATION

Robert Snowden, BA, PhD, DSA, is Professor of Family Studies in the Sociology Department of the University of Exeter, and previously founder-director of the Institute of Population Studies, University of Exeter. Currently a member of the Human Fertilisation and Embryology Authority and Chairman of the Medical Editorial Advisory Panel of the International Planned Parenthood Federation, he is also an Honorary Life Member of the Family Planning Association and Chairman of Exeter Relate.

Elizabeth Snowden, BEd, SRN, is Research Assistant in the Institute of Population Studies, University of Exeter. She is a founder-member of the British Infertility Counselling Association, an Honorary Life Member of the Family Planning Association and a trustee of the Margaret Jackson Trust.

Robert and Elizabeth Snowden have worked together over many years in support of those who wish to plan their families in the most acceptable and efficient way. They have published widely on subjects relating to the planning of families.

THE GIFT OF A CHILD

From reviews of this new edition:

Many couples seeking DI feel that they are walking alone through a minefield. They are desperate to consult others who have trodden the path before ... this book is invaluable to them. It investigates both the causes of male infertility and the complex issues behind DI. It tries hard to provide answers using extracts from interviews with couples who have undergone, and in many cases have children as a result of, DI. These frank and often emotional dialogues are of great comfort to the reader.

ISSUE Newsletter

First published and given 'FPA approval' in 1984, it is excellent to see a new edition of this helpful publication ... The book comprehensively covers the physical, emotional, legal and ethical implications of donor insemination by drawing on the collective experiences of couples who achieved a family in this way. It is a valuable, informative book.

Toni Belfield, Head of Information and Research,
Family Planning Association

The book has been very well received by our members, and has proven to be a great help to them.

Caroline Stone, Vice-Chair CHILD

The Gift of a Child

A GUIDE TO DONOR INSEMINATION

SECOND REVISED EDITION

Robert and Elizabeth Snowden

UNIVERSITY
of
EXETER
PRESS

First published by George Allen & Unwin in 1984.

Second edition first published in 1993 by

University of Exeter Press
Reed Hall, Streatham Drive
Exeter, Devon
EX4 4QR
UK

Reprinted 1994

British Library Cataloguing in Publication Data
A catalogue record for this book
is available from the British Library

ISBN 0 85989 407 X

Typeset in 11/12.5 Palatino by Exe Valley Dataset Ltd, Exeter
Printed and bound in Great Britain by BPC Wheatons Ltd, Exeter

Contents

In memory of Margaret Jackson, a much loved pioneer in the provision of family planning and infertility treatment; and of Muriel Bartlett, without whose help Margaret would not have been able to achieve so much in her tireless efforts to improve the quality of life for so many women.

Foreword to the Revised Edition

This book has been written in fulfilment of a promise made to couples, individuals, parents and children who have been willing to describe their experiences resulting from their participation in the particular form of infertility treatment known as donor insemination. We were asked to share this experience with the aim of helping the thousands of childless couples who might be considering donor insemination as a way of dealing with their childlessness. We have kept in touch with many of these families and have been privileged to be invited into their homes to discuss the developing relationships between the parents and their specially conceived children. In many respects this is their story and we gratefully acknowledge the part they have played in it.

The first edition of this book was published in 1984 and since then a great deal has changed in relation to the provision of donor insemination as an infertility treatment. Numerous committees, working groups and official consultations have taken place resulting in legislation, the Human Fertilisation and Embryology Act 1990, which governs this and other types of treatment in which donated sperm or eggs are used. Since 1984 there has also been a steady growth in the membership of self-help groups such as 'Issue' (The National Fertility Association) and 'Child'. During this period a second round of interviews has also taken place among the families whom we first met in 1980 and a further sharing of information has taken place about family experiences now that the children have started secondary school.

We have also been involved in official study groups and informal working parties during this period, as new regulations and laws have been formulated to deal with the growing provision of donor insemination services. This has allowed us to link the public issues described in official reports to the more personal concerns of couples and individuals whose lives are deeply affected by infertility, childlessness and the provision of treatment services.

Alongside the families who have co-operated with us have been the staff of such organisations as the King's Fund, the Human Fertilisation and Embryology Authority (HFEA), the Institute of Population Studies and the Sociology Department in Exeter University. Helpful advice has been provided by 'Issue', 'Child', the Fertility Committee of the Royal College of Obstetricians & Gynaecologists and by members of the British Infertility Counselling Association. Dr Sheila Cook provided up-dated information about the practicalities of donor insemination treatment. Professor Duncan Mitchell has been a valuable member of the research team and helped with many of the interviews. Secretarial support has been provided by Mrs Mary Guy and the original research was undertaken using financial support provided by the Economic & Social Research Council.

We thank you all.

Robert and Elizabeth Snowden
Exeter University, 1993.

Introduction

The experience of infertility is much more common than most people realise. In Britain about 400,000 couples get married or set up house together each year. When these couples decide to have children over 40,000 of them will find they are unable to start a family. In about 16,000 of these couples the cause of the infertility will lie with the man, in a similar number with the woman, and in a further 8,000 couples both male and female partners may have contributing factors.

There is a mistaken belief that infertility is a woman's problem only and it comes as a great surprise to many people that a man, certainly a man capable of enjoying sexual activity and having normal sexual feelings, can be infertile. Most people imagine that infertility must mean impotence and that a man who is virile and capable of enjoying sexual activity must be fertile. But fertility and virility are quite different things. It is entirely possible for a man who is virile and physically sexually competent to produce semen that has little or no fertilising capacity.

Because infertility is generally thought to be a woman's problem, most books for the infertile couple are addressed to a predominantly female audience and concentrate on female forms of infertility and infertility treatment. The experience and treatment of men who are infertile is virtually ignored, or at best discussed briefly, and couples often search in vain for adequate information. To want children and to be unable to have them causes much heart-break for men and women alike; the pain of childlessness would be difficult to exaggerate. If couples are to be helped to deal with this crisis in their lives they need adequate information about infertility and an opportunity to examine their own feelings about it. Understanding a problem is half-way towards resolving it.

In this book we attempt to explain what male infertility is and to explore the feelings which infertile couples often experience. We also discuss alternative ways and means of solving the problem of involuntary childlessness, concentrating particularly on some of the more common questions which are asked about donor insemination (DI). This procedure used to be known as artificial insemination by donor (or AID) but the name was changed in order to avoid confusion with the disease of AIDS. Donor insemination is a procedure which is not easily discussed by couples where the male partner is found to be infertile. This means that each couple faces the problem anew and in isolation; couples are often unable to benefit from the knowledge and experience of others who have found themselves in a similar situation. This book seeks to support a more open attitude towards DI, and to pass on the collective experience of many couples who have achieved a family by means of DI to those couples (and their advisers) who are newly confronting the problem of male infertility.

It is not possible to give hard-and-fast, factual answers to most questions about DI. Most questions presented in this book are discussed rather than answered by drawing on the experience of the many parents with whom we talked during our researches. Of course their experience is not all the same and their opinions often differ. Nevertheless it is possible to examine their experiences and their opinions and to draw out from these common themes, patterns of similar problems and ways of dealing with them. These parents of children conceived by DI allowed us into their homes, and gave their time to answer very intimate and personal questions, and shared painful as well as happy memories with us. We hope they will feel they have been repaid if their experience can be used to help other couples avoid some of the pitfalls, and to come to well-founded decisions in their efforts to find a solution to their childlessness.

1

Male Infertility

The prevalence of male infertility

Most people assume that male infertility is extremely rare and uncommon. If a couple is having difficulty in starting a baby, this difficulty is usually assumed to be due to some condition affecting the woman. Indeed, until fairly recently, if a couple went to consult their doctor about their difficulty in not being able to get pregnant it was the woman who was examined first. It was not until she had been subjected to an exhaustive (and exhausting) battery of tests without discovering any reason for her inability to have a baby that tests were then carried out on her male partner. This practice of investigating the woman first would seem to give credence to the idea that infertility must be primarily a woman's problem and that male infertility must be rare.

This lack of awareness of the fairly common incidence of male infertility means that when a man learns he is infertile he also has the additional problem of feeling that he alone has been singled out for this calamity. One wife said to us during an interview: 'When we were first told about it we thought we were unique cases, because you don't realise how common it is.'

Not only is the condition of infertility hard to accept, news of it also has the psychological effect of marking the infertile man off from other men and he often feels isolated and alone. It is not surprising that men should think they are unique cases; this is because they almost never hear of any other cases happening among their friends and relatives when it is discovered that they are infertile. Many men feel (quite wrongly) that their virility and their manliness is being called into question; so it is to some extent understandable that most men do not talk openly about their infertility. Their partners also very often help to keep it all quiet by sometimes going so far as to pretend that it is they who are the infertile partner. For a woman to admit to infertility is believed to be more acceptable than for a man openly to admit to this condition. But all this has the grave disadvantage of giving a false picture and it is not surprising that each new man who learns he is infertile thinks he is the only one so afflicted. In addition, if people in general are never given the opportunity to hear and learn about male infertility, they will never have the opportunity to discover their misconceptions about the subject and to become more informed and understanding.

Let us consider how rare, or rather how common, male infertility really is. It is generally accepted that about 10 per cent of all couples will have difficulty in starting a family when they decide to do so. In Britain just under 400,000 couples get married or set up house together each year, so if 10 per cent of couples experience some degree of infertility this means that each year 40,000 couples in Britain will find that they are unable to achieve a pregnancy when they want to. The source of the infertility is fairly evenly divided between men and women. In about 40 per cent of the cases the woman will have some degree of infertility, and in about 40 per cent of cases it will be the man who is affected. In the remaining 20 per cent of cases it will either not be possible to establish any definite reason for infertility, or it will be due to joint factors in both partners. This means that every year in Britain approximately 16,000 men will experience infertility or sub-fertility; and in a further 8,000 couples the male partner may be contributing to the infertility. The next time a couple experiencing male infertility encounter a large group of people—say on a Saturday morning shopping trip—it is worth considering that on average, every tenth couple met is likely to have experienced problems when they wanted a baby and that one in every 25 couples will have a problem relating to male infertility. Knowledge of this relatively common incidence of infertility can provide affected men with some solace in their discomfort. Knowledge that there are many other men in a similar position often brings with it a sense of shared experience. This is important because it usually provides a sense of relief and helps to restore confidence. Though the infertility is still distressing, at least the man no longer needs to feel an isolated and unique oddity. During our research, couples whom we visited were surprised and gratified to learn how many other couples were involved in the research. The comment of one man is typical of many: 'It's nice to know you're not the only person. I didn't realise there were so many.' Just knowing that there are other people in a similar position is important irrespective of whether or not medical treatment is sought.

There are many causes of male infertility and in order to understand how such infertility comes about, it is necessary first to have some basic knowledge of the workings of the male reproductive system.

The male reproductive system

It is at puberty, usually at about the age of 12 years, that the male reproductive system becomes functional. Before that age the system remains dormant. The production of sperm begins in the testes, stimulated by messages carried in the bloodstream in the form of hormones from a special gland situated in the base of the brain—the pituitary gland. These gonadotrophic hormones as they are called travel to the testes and stimulate them to begin production of another hormone called testosterone. It is testosterone which is the male sex hormone. Not only does it play a part in the production of sperm, but it is also responsible for changes in the body which become the outward signs of puberty; for example, the growth of hair on the face, under the arms and in the pubic region. Other hormones are also involved which, with the gonadotrophic hormones and testosterone, work together in a delicately balanced way to control sperm production. Some of the hormones act as a kind of switch mechanism which turns on (or turns off) the production of other hormones to maintain this delicate balance. Any disruption of this very delicate balance of hormones may interfere with sperm development and eventually lead to infertility. Normally, once sperm production commences it continues throughout a man's adult life.

The *testes* are two small oval glands situated in the *scrotum* which is a pouch of skin lying outside the body. The testes are initially formed inside the abdomen during the period of development before birth. Shortly before birth the two testes descend into the scrotum to lie outside the main body cavity. This ensures a slightly lower temperature within the testes and this reduced temperature is a necessary condition for satisfactory sperm production.

Sperm (or *Spermatozoa*) are produced in the testes; this production is a continuous and very complex process in which immature cells gradually develop over a period of ten or eleven weeks into mature sperm. A layer of cells known as the *germinal epithelium* produces the cells from which each sperm develops. If this layer of germinal epithelium is damaged or destroyed there is no raw material for sperm development. Mature sperm are tadpole-shaped with a head and tail and are very small indeed. They are about 2,000 times smaller than the woman's egg (or *ovum*) which is just visible to the naked eye. Each sperm contains chromosomes (including the one which will determine the sex of the child) which combine with the chromosomes of the ovum when fertilisation occurs. Together these chromosomes contain all the ingredients which will provide the distinctive and unique inherited characteristics of the child to be born. Sperm are produced in vast numbers; on average anything up to 400

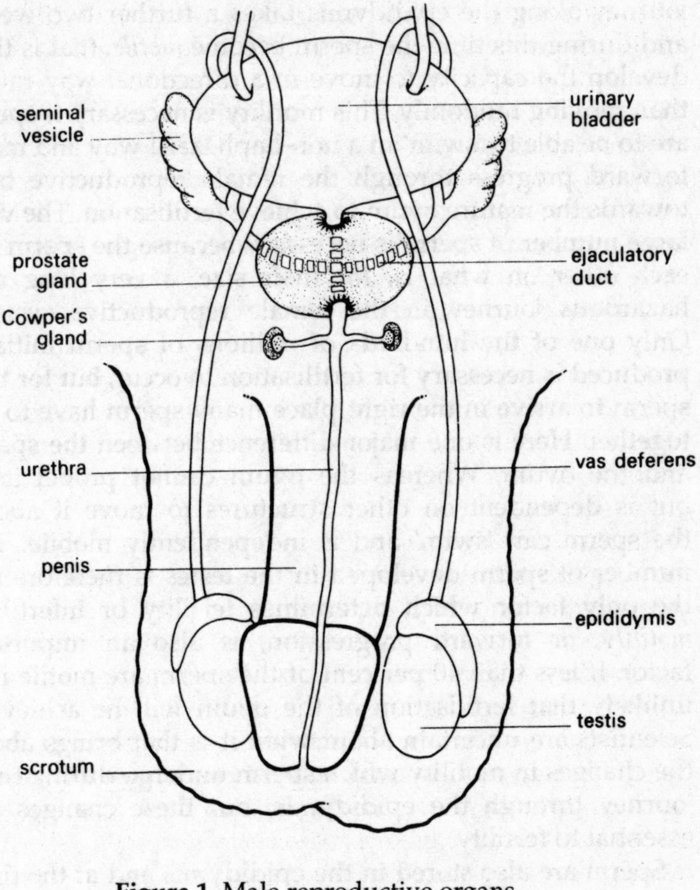

Figure 1. Male reproductive organs

million sperm are ejaculated at each orgasm. It is usual for some of the sperm to be imperfectly formed and to show some abnormality in their shape or *morphology*. However if many of the sperm are abnormally formed it reduces the likelihood that fertilisation of the ovum will occur.

After development sperm leave each testis and travel into a fine coiled tube known as the *epididymis* which lies adjacent to the testis. This fine tube would be about six metres long if it was unravelled and stretched out. The journey along the epididymis takes a further two weeks and during this time the sperm become *motile*, that is they develop the capacity to move in a directional way rather than moving randomly. This motility is necessary if sperm are to be able to 'swim' in a non-haphazard way and make forward progress through the female reproductive tract towards the mature ovum to achieve fertilisation. The very large number of sperm is necessary because the sperm aid each other on what is, for their size, a very long and hazardous journey in the female reproductive system. Only one of the hundreds of millions of sperm initially produced is necessary for fertilisation to occur, but for that sperm to arrive in the right place many sperm have to act together. Here is one major difference between the sperm and the ovum. Whereas the ovum cannot propel itself but is dependent on other structures to move it about, the sperm can 'swim' and is independently mobile. The number of sperm developed in the testes is therefore not the only factor which determines fertility or infertility; *motility*, or forward progression, is also an important factor. If less than 40 per cent of the sperm are motile it is unlikely that fertilisation of the ovum will be achieved. Scientists are uncertain about what it is that brings about the changes in motility which sperm undergo during their journey through the epididymis, but these changes are essential to fertility.

Sperm are also stored in the epididymis and at the time of ejaculation they leave the epididymis and pass along a tube, the *vas deferens* (this is the tube which is sealed off in a vasectomy operation), and into the ejaculatory ducts and urethra. During this journey, secretions from three sets of glands help to transport the sperm. These glands (known as the seminal vesicles, Cowper's glands and the prostate gland—see Figure 1) contribute the thick, milky substance which is visible at ejaculation, the sperm themselves being too small to see. This *seminal fluid* must be of the correct consistency and composition if the sperm is to achieve its objective of fertilising the ovum. The seminal fluid together with the sperm is known as *semen* and at the time of ejaculation about one teaspoonful (between 2 and 5 millilitres) is produced. In order to ensure that this semen, which contains anything up to 400 million sperm, is placed deep inside the female reproductive system, the penis has to be in an erect state. Erection is governed by nerve impulses which dilate certain blood vessels and constrict others in the penis allowing the erectile tissue to fill with blood. While the penis is in the erect condition ejaculation can occur. There are really two processes taking place here; first, the sperm have to be moved from the storage place in the epididymis, along the vas deferens, through the ejaculatory ducts and into the urethra. This phase is called *emission*. Second, once in the urethra the semen is violently driven along the urethra and out of the erect penis by means of a powerful contraction of muscles in the penis itself and those attached to the urethra. This is called *ejaculation* and is normally accompanied by male orgasm.

At this point the male role in reproduction is over, although many millions of sperm are beginning what is a very long and hazardous journey for them. It only takes one of these millions of sperm to effect a pregnancy. However, conception is never certain, for fertilisation can only take place during a very brief period in the female monthly menstrual cycle; the timing has to be just right.

The causes of male infertility

There are three main ways in which male fertility may be impaired:

(i) certain factors may prevent or adversely affect the production and maturation of sperm;

(ii) blockages in the ducts and channels of the male reproductive organs may prevent sperm which are produced from getting into the seminal fluid which is ejaculated at orgasm;

(iii) certain conditions may prevent the normal delivery of the semen into the vagina during sexual intercourse.

It has been estimated that only in about one-half of the cases of male infertility can a specific cause for the infertility be found. In the other half of cases the cause remains a mystery. Where no cause can be identified the infertility is termed *idiopathic*.

Semen capable of effecting a pregnancy contains anything from 20 million to over 100 million sperm per millilitre. If semen contains less than 20 million sperm in each millilitre this condition is known as *oligospermia* (literally 'few sperm') and it is unlikely that such semen would be successful in starting a pregnancy. Sometimes, if the female partner is extremely fertile this may compensate for the reduced fertility of the male and conception might occur, but the likelihood is greatly reduced. If there is a complete absence of sperm from the semen, this condition is known as *azoospermia* (literally 'no sperm'). In such cases it is impossible for the semen to bring about a conception and pregnancy.

Perhaps the most well-known cause of male infertility is *mumps*. The virus which causes mumps usually infects the salivary glands which are situated at the side of the face, but sometimes if an adult male contracts mumps, the virus may also infect the testes causing a condition known as *orchitis*. This infection damages the layer of cells in the testes which would normally develop into mature sperm, with the result that these cells are no longer capable of developing.

Other viral infections which cause a high fever, such as glandular fever or infective hepatitis, may also interfere with sperm production for a time, but usually the basic cells are not destroyed completely and recovery of function returns within a few months.

Another important cause of male infertility is the presence of a *varicocele*. This is a kind of varicose vein of the testicle and may be large or small. The enlarged vein is caused by a reflux of blood coming from the renal vein, a vein which serves the kidney. Not all men who have a varicocele are infertile, and it is still not completely clear just how a varicocele causes infertility. There are two possible explanations. The increased volume of blood present may cause an increase in the temperature within the scrotum and so interfere with sperm production. Alternatively it is thought that it may be the concentration of toxic substances which are present in the blood of the renal vein which damages the tissue of the testis and impairs sperm production. In some cases it is possible to improve fertility by an operation in which the affected 'varicose' vein is tied or blocked off in some way.

Increased heat may also cause a reduction in fertility. The testes function at a temperature almost 2° C lower than body temperature. This lower temperature is achieved because the testes are situated in the scrotum, outside the abdominal cavity. If tight underpants or tight jeans are worn, these press the testes against the body and the scrotal temperature may rise. Athletic supports or protective boxes worn in certain sports may also cause an increase in scrotal temperature. By simply wearing more loosely fitting clothes and bathing the scrotum with cold water once or twice daily, fertility can sometimes be improved.

Undescended testicles are another important cause of male infertility. Before birth, during the development of the foetus, the testes are initially formed within the abdominal cavity. Only later in foetal development, in the final weeks before the baby is born, do they descend into the scrotal cavity. Sometimes one or both testes fail to descend in the normal way and remain within the abdominal cavity. This condition is known as *cryptorchidism*. If this condition is left untreated it is associated with azoospermia. Damage to the undescended testes will occur—almost certainly by the age of 3 years—and becomes progressively worse the longer the testes remain within the abdominal cavity. This damage is irreversible and interferes with sperm production. The testes can be surgically brought down into the scrotal sac, in an operation called *orchidopexy*, and this stops any further damage being done but does not counter the damage which has already occurred. Doctors are not in complete agreement about the best age for this operation to be carried out. One might think 'the earlier the better', but operations on babies or very tiny children are difficult and most doctors advise that the operation is best left until the child is between 5 and 8 years of age.

Disorders affecting endocrine glands, such as the pituitary, the thyroid or the adrenal glands, may also cause male infertility. The hormones produced by endocrine glands work together in a very complex and finely balanced system and if this balance is upset sperm production may be impaired. However, hormone disorders are not a common cause of male infertility and it has been estimated that only 10 per cent of cases are caused by hormone deficiency or imbalance.

Genetic disorders are another rare cause of male infertility. In these cases the information which is stored in the chromosomes and genes, and which determines the construction of body tissues and substances, is faulty. One such example is *Klinefelter's syndrome* which accounts for 1–2 per cent of cases of male infertility. Normally a pair of chromosomes, known as the XY chromosomes provide the basis for the male sex of a child. In Klinefelter's syndrome an extra chromosome is present, an additional X chromosome, making XXY. This additional X chromosome causes changes throughout the male child's body and is associated with azoospermia.

Radiation, either encountered accidentally during employment or used in the treatment of a malignant disease, may also impair or stop sperm production. Damage to the testes may also result from the use of drugs, particularly the cyto-toxic drugs used in the treatment of malignancy or from immunosuppressive drugs used to prevent tissue rejection. Exposure to some chemical compounds used in industrial processes or in agriculture may also cause infertility.

Infertility may also result as a complication of other diseases such as renal failure or untreated diabetes. Smoking, excessive alcohol consumption, stress, malnutrition and obesity are all factors which it is thought may contribute to a reduction of fertility.

Infections such as gonorrhoea, or more rarely tuberculosis, may cause inflammation and blockage of the vas deferens or the ejaculatory ducts. Infection may also cause blockage of the finely coiled tube of the epididymis and prevent the passage of sperm. These infections may be difficult to diagnose and stubborn to treat. Rarely there may be a congenital absence of a part of the system of tubes and ducts which fails to develop, and so the ducts do not connect up into one continuous channel.

Failure to deliver semen into the vagina during sexual intercourse may be due to impotence. Impotence may be caused by psychological factors or may be due to organic disease such as diabetes. Certain drugs, for example those used in the treatment of raised blood pressure, may have the side effect of impotence. Faulty delivery of sperm may also be caused by disorders of ejaculation. Ejaculation is a reflex action which is controlled by a complex sequence of nerve impulses. Sometimes, following spinal injury or surgery to the bladder or rectum, these nerve pathways which control the process of ejaculation may be damaged. In these cases ejaculation may not occur at all, or semen may be expelled in the wrong direction into the bladder—a condition known as *retrograde ejaculation*.

Semen analysis

The fertility of semen can be assessed by microscopic examination. This is usually done on two occasions about a month apart because results for the same man can vary on different occasions. The laboratory carrying out the test will give clear instructions about the collection of the sample and delivery to the laboratory; these must be followed carefully, otherwise it is possible that the semen might deteriorate before examination is complete. The semen will be examined in terms of its total amount, the number and concentration of sperm it contains, as well as their activity (*motility*) and structure (*morphology*). The laboratory will report any other findings thought to be of relevance, and taking all these measures into consideration together, the specialist will assess the overall fertilising capacity of the semen sample.

Research into male infertility

Research into the causes and the treatment of male infertility has had some successes, but in the main the results of this research have been disappointing. Various reasons for this failure to achieve a successful breakthrough have been suggested. Traditionally infertility has been seen as a woman's problem and so research expertise and funding have been concentrated on infertility in women. The medical speciality of gynaecology, dealing with disease and malfunction of the female reproductive system, is well established. However until recently there has been no comparable separate specialism dealing with the male reproductive system. Investigation of male infertility was usually undertaken by urologists, that is, specialists in the combined fields of genito-urinary diseases, because of the common organs involved. But clearly the study of male infertility has little to do with the study of urinary disease, and for most urologists the detailed study of male infertility has not been their primary interest.

The fact that there was no specialism entirely devoted to the study of male infertility had a detrimental effect on the progress of research. The processes whereby healthy sperm are produced are very complex and are still not fully understood. For example, very little is known about the changes which confer the capacity for motility on the sperm during their passage through and their subsequent storage in the epididymis. However, the specialism of *andrology* has now been established to study reproduction and fertility in the male and there are signs that the problems of male infertility are now beginning to receive more determined attention from researchers.

One recent discovery is that a substance called *Pentoxifylline* can improve the motility of defective sperm and thus improve its fertilising capacity. Recent research in Australia using Pentoxyfylline has produced some encouraging results. Research is also being undertaken to help treatment in cases where azoospermia is due to a blockage in or absence of the duct system. An operation, under general anaesthetic, to collect sperm directly from the epididymis is now being developed.

For men whose semen analysis shows some sperm, but of insufficient concentration or motility to make natural conception likely, the new *in-vitro* fertilisation techniques of assisted conception (popularly called test-tube-baby techniques) also hold out a degree of hope by allowing the infertility specialist to make the best use of the sperm there are. However, these new options are at an early stage of development, have a high failure rate and are not available to men suffering from a complete absence of sperm.

One of the main reasons why treatment of male infertility is often not possible or not successful, is because in as many as one-half of all cases the cause of the infertility cannot be determined. If the cause is not known, obviously treatment becomes difficult. Another reason for disappointing results of treatment is that damage to the testes is often irreversible. After puberty sperm production is a continuous process and normally sperm are developing throughout a man's adult life. But if the basic cells which form the raw material have already been destroyed sperm production cannot occur even though the conditions are subsequently more favourable.

In some ways the availability of DI may also have played a part in diverting attention away from seeking a cure for male infertility. DI does nothing to cure a man's infertility, but it does circumvent it and allow him to become the father of children. DI can be used without the knowledge of others; this combined with the wish by most infertile men to avoid making their infertility known means that there has been little demand from these men for closer attention to their problems and for the encouragement of relevant research. While men remain unwilling to admit that infertility is a condition which affects men as frequently as it affects women, male infertility is unlikely to receive the energetic research attention it needs and deserves.

2

Childlessness

Voluntary and involuntary childlessness

It should not be assumed that childlessness is always due to infertility. It is becoming increasingly common for couples to elect not to have children, to make a positive decision to remain child-free. Such *voluntary* childlessness is the result of a purposeful decision by the couple and results in a situation which is quite different from *involuntary* childlessness. When a couple decide that they do want children, and then find that this decision is thwarted, such involuntary childlessness becomes a very distressing, frustrating and sometimes destructive condition. The heart-ache of couples who want to start a family of their own and who are unable to do so is very real and can cast a shadow over their whole lives. This distress cannot be exaggerated and the knowledge that a large number of other couples are similarly afflicted may alleviate some of the feelings of isolation, but the pain nevertheless remains.

This distinction between voluntary and involuntary childlessness is, however, not always as clear-cut a distinction as it may first appear. Sometimes a couple who want children and who are able to conceive a child of their own decide to forgo the option of having their own baby. For example, it may be inadvisable for a couple to have a child because of the possibility that one or both of them may pass on to the child an hereditary disease or disability. It is possible, where there is a suspicion that an hereditary disorder is present, for couples to obtain specialist advice from a genetic counsellor about the risk of having an affected child. Such help is needed by few couples, but it is freely available as part of the National Health Service and can be arranged by the family doctor. Here is a situation which is especially painful for the couple who would like to have a child of their own. They are able to conceive but to attempt a pregnancy would be unwise. The distress such couples must experience in coming to a 'voluntary' decision not to have a child can hardly be imagined.

One reason why a couple may be unable to conceive a child may be that the man has previously undergone a vasectomy operation in order to have a more permanent method of contraception once he and his partner have had the number of children they want. The couple may later regret this decision and decide they want another child. More commonly a vasectomised man who has children by a previous partner from whom he is now separated or divorced may wish to have children with his new partner. Some surgeons do attempt an operation to reverse the effects of vasectomy, but on the whole the results are disappointing. Even if the *vas deferens* can be refashioned into a continuous hollow tube again, the ability to father children often does not return.

These examples indicate that there is a considerable overlap between what we have called involuntary and voluntary childlessness. It is hard to say which is worse for the couple: clear knowledge that a pregnancy is not possible, or where a pregnancy is possible but unwise, or where a pregnancy is possible but someone else's sperm is used. The experience of infertility can leave little or no room for choice or it can provide an agonising choice. In whatever form it is presented, the unhappiness it causes is often similar and cannot be denied.

The experience of infertility

Most couples expect to have children in the natural run of events; the setting up of a home and the birth of children are usually seen as going together. The only decision most couples think they have to make is to decide when to start having a family. Few think of the possibility of infertility, so to learn that one is not fertile usually comes as a great shock. One woman with whom we were discussing these things said to her husband: 'It was a shock that you haven't really got over, wasn't it? Both of us really. Because you don't expect it—not yourself—not really.' Not only is it a shock, but it is a shock that often leaves a man feeling inadequate, and somehow less of a man. Her husband replied: 'I felt, well, a bit useless at the time.' Another man described his reactions on being told that he was infertile: 'Anyone who's never actually been told, you can't tell them the feeling that you get. It's like being hit with a sledge-hammer . . . . I never felt so ill in my life. It took me a long while to get over it.'

A major part of this shock of infertility is caused because many men feel it casts doubts on their masculinity, on their manhood. One man we talked with said: 'If you tell most people you are sterile they think you are not virile and you can be jibed about it and people just don't understand.' This man had not actually told anyone, but he was sure that this would be the reaction. Of course, if a man feels his masculinity and virility have been called into question, this anxiety of itself can trigger problems with sexual performance. One American doctor who studied the reactions of men who had just been told of their infertility found that almost two-thirds of them had experienced a brief period of impotence lasting for one to three months following the discovery. Fortunately in most cases this difficulty was short-lived and sexual potency was recovered as the couple gradually adjusted to the new situation.

But of course fertility is not the same thing as virility. One partner of an infertile man we interviewed noted the difference and said about infertile men: 'They are men in every sense of the word, they still make love, they are masculine and everything.' Those who have first-hand experience of male infertility know this to be true, but because infertile men generally feel the need to hide their infertility from others, the prejudices most people hold about infertility are not challenged. It is certainly true that most couples feel it is more socially acceptable for a woman to say she is infertile than it is for a man to admit to his infertility. It is common for women to pretend that it is they, and not their partner, who are infertile. If couples are to understand their own feelings about infertility, these prejudices about male infertility need to be examined more closely; they have much to do with stereotypical images about appropriate behaviour. The male is expected to take the initiative, to be strong, to achieve and to succeed. In the event of initial failure he must persevere and persist until he does succeed, and it is considered a weakness for him to fail or to show his feelings of distress if success eludes him. Infertility in a man conflicts with this stereotype of the masculine image. He may feel he has to hide his grief and emotions and deny what he may see as his 'failure' if he is to maintain his masculine image. On the other hand the stereotypical woman belongs to the 'weaker sex' and is expected to show her emotions. So a woman can admit to infertility without sacrificing anything of her feminine image. In recent years most men and women have begun to examine the behaviour and roles which have been unthinkingly expected of them. Whilst the feminist movement and the pressure for women to challenge masculine values may have caught the headlines, there has also been a realisation that men's lives may be enriched by sharing in what have been formerly regarded as feminine values. Men, as well as women, need to be able to admit their inner feelings of grief. Men, too, benefit from the release of emotion and tension which acknowledging these very natural feelings brings. It is not a failing in a man to have deep feelings of hurt and disappointment and to be willing to acknowledge these.

However, infertility means more than just a possible threat to a man's masculinity; it means that a man cannot procreate children of his own who will continue his ancestral line. Children represent a continuity of the past, present and the future; they provide the means by which parents can live on in future generations. When asked about his feelings concerning his own infertility, one man said to us:

> My major hang-up really was based on this rather metaphysical notion of genetic immortality. What depressed me most of all, and overwhelmed me mentally, was this idea that at this point my genetic channel stops. That's the end. And that was the most chilling thing I had to take on board.

The problem of 'genetic death' for the infertile male is of course not solved by his wife having a baby through the use of someone else's sperm, as in the case of DI. DI does not cure a man's infertility, it circumvents his childlessness by allowing him to nurture a child who is genetically linked to his partner but who is not genetically linked to himself. This same man, who was the father of two DI children, also said:

> I must be frank and say that I still wish that I could father a child; this is still a faint note of sadness to me. But it doesn't intrude into my relationship with these two children, because I can really put my hand on my heart and say I wouldn't really change them. But I think if somebody suddenly discovered that my fertility had come back I would want to try most vigorously to have a child. But I think that's a very primeval and natural response.

Although a woman who's partner is infertile does not share her partner's infertility, she does share his childlessness. One woman in this position said to us:

> When I was holding someone's baby, or even looking after little children, I'd play with them and do all sorts and it was lovely. But when I went home, I could have climbed up the wall because there was so much love inside of me that I couldn't give.

Many women experience spontaneous feelings of anger and resentment that their partner cannot give them children. These feelings are common and quite natural, but the woman may feel guilty and ashamed at having these thoughts, and find it hard to acknowledge that they feel such things about their partner.

Several husbands we talked with admitted that when they first became aware of their infertility, they had offered their wife a divorce because they could not give her children. They said they did this because they felt they were not able to meet their obligations to the marriage. These obligations are rarely made explicit but nevertheless remain unspoken assumptions that a husband should be able to give his wife a child. Many infertile men feel this sense of inadequacy very strongly. The man believes he has let his partner down in not being able to fulfil the role he feels his partner expects of him. He thinks the least he can do is to offer his partner the opportunity of release from a partnership which cannot give what she has a right to expect. While this reaction is understandable, it has to be remembered that having children is only one aspect of a couple's relationship. Most women wish for a child as the result of a loving relationship and such a relationship is more than the ability to produce children. Perhaps the offer of a divorce or separation is more of a cry for help at a time of stress and anguish. If couples can admit to these painful, contradictory and sometimes destructive emotions which are quite natural and experienced by virtually all couples when infertility is first diagnosed, the first step has been taken towards adjustment to their inability to have children in the usual way.

Nevertheless the frustration of the desire to have children is extremely distressing and many couples with whom we talked about their infertility expressed the view that those who have children without difficulty could never understand the heartache suffered by childless couples in their efforts to have children. In some respects the possibility of successful treatment offered by recent scientific advances has actually increased the stress experienced by childless couples. Before these new possibilities of treatment were available couples had no alternative but to accept their lot; now couples may feel personally at fault if they do not pursue every possibility, however remote and costly, in their efforts to overcome their inability to have children.

However treatment is not always possible or successful. If a couple are to come to terms with their involuntary childlessness, and if a man is to come to terms successfully with his infertility, they must be able to acknowledge the reality of the situation. It is here that the help of a skilled independent counsellor can be invaluable. A counsellor cannot provide ready made answers to a couple's problems but he or she can enable couples to explore and understand their feelings better so that they themselves can see their own situation more clearly. The couple can then come to more appropriate decisions about what their course of action should be. This acceptance of a new and difficult situation may take some time, and both partners may well experience painful feelings of disbelief, anger, guilt and depression. But it is essential that the situation is faced honestly and openly, however painful this may be. In some respects news of infertility and childlessness is like suffering a bereavement. Infertility means the loss of a child which the couple had planned, even though it is the loss of a child who never came into being. Couples may feel intense grief at their awareness of this loss. It is natural to feel this grief, and it is helpful to allow oneself to grieve and to go through a time of mourning. In time this process of grieving helps to reduce and accept this sense of loss and eventually one is able to look forward to life again in a more constructive way. Once a couple have faced up to and accepted the fact that they are not going to be able to have a child of their own in the usual way, they can begin to make new decisions about future plans. They can discuss and work out together what is, for them, the best possible alternative course of action.

The resolution of childlessness

There are three main options open to childless couples where the male partner is infertile. They can decide to remain child-free; they can approach an adoption agency or they can consider donor insemination. In a very few cases a fourth more experimental option exists when infertility is due to oligospermia. Using the procedure of external *in-vitro* fertilisation it is occasionally possible to select out individual sperm and, using microscopic techniques, to assist the sperm to penetrate the coating of the ovum so that fertilisation occurs.

Remaining childfree

Remaining childfree may seem a strange option to discuss—really not an alternative at all. Couples might be wise to take time to discuss with each other and to think out just why they decided they wanted to have children in the first place. Indeed, did they ever actually *decide* at all, or was it something that they just took for granted. As we said earlier, having children tends to be seen as the natural thing to do and there is considerable pressure on couples to conform to this way of life. Perhaps a couple may find that once they have settled and established a home their parents, other relatives and even friends, begin to drop hints about the expected arrival of a baby. Or perhaps a couple's friends have had children and the couple may be made to feel a bit 'left behind'. Often a couple may not be conscious of these pressures to have children which sometimes take very subtle forms. But increasingly people, particularly young people, are beginning to question the 'naturalness' of having children. Some of them are beginning to realise that perhaps their wish for children merely reflects what is expected of them, and is not really a matter of personal choice. Efficient contraception means that fertile couples can now consciously decide that they would prefer to remain child-free; and this permits them to channel their energies and their creativity into other activities which, if they had children, they would not have the freedom to pursue.

Similarly some infertile couples may find, when they think about it, that perhaps they were going to have children only because it was expected of them and not because it was something that they really wanted for themselves. Such couples might after all prefer to live as a couple without children. What the diagnosis of infertility has done in such cases is to remove the element of choice, and to come to terms with this restriction is not the same as having to come to terms with infertility itself. In all seriousness, the advantages and disadvantages of remaining child-free should be the first consideration of couples where one of the partners is infertile.

One last word of caution; remaining child-free is an option that is different from seeking adoption, donor insemination, or the even more technical forms of assisted conception. Provided age is not a limiting factor, the decision to remain child-free can always be reversed by seeking these other alternatives at a later date. A rush to deal with childlessness following news of infertility is unwise. Couples should give themselves time to think this issue through carefully and thoughtfully. Remaining child-free can be a temporary condition. We have already described the possible strain on a relationship when male infertility is first discovered. The extreme forms of this stress—impotency and the offer of divorce or separation—are often temporary. A decision concerning what to do about childlessness should at least be delayed for a few months to ensure that it is really a child that is wanted and not relief from such disagreeable, but temporary, experiences. Remaining child-free should be the situation of choice—at least for a time.

Adoption

For many years adoption has been the usual way in which infertile couples have solved their problem of childlessness. If there is a baby unable to be looked after by its natural parents and an infertile couple who want a baby but are unable to have one of their own, it seems sensible to attempt to solve both problems by the same means. Over the years a framework of laws and legal procedures has been established to regulate the process of adoption. This legal framework protects the needs and the rights of the child and also safeguards the rights of the natural and the adoptive parents. Adoptions are arranged either by officially registered adoption agencies or by local authority social service departments. When a couple apply to become adoptive parents they are visited by a social worker who will try to assess if the couple and their home are suitable. If accepted, the couple will be placed on a waiting list until a baby who is thought to be suitable for them is in need of adoptive parents. The adoption procedure is lengthy and can be stressful for all concerned. No legal steps can be taken before the baby is 6 weeks old. This gives the natural mother time to think out the alternatives carefully and to make up her mind whether or not adoption is the best thing for her baby and for herself. After this period of six weeks, and if the natural mother has decided to go ahead with adoption, prospective adoptive parents can apply for an adoption order. It is usually at least three months before this order is granted. Until then the natural mother may, if she changes her mind, apply to the court to withdraw her agreement to adoption. During this time a temporary guardian (called a guardian *ad litem*) is appointed to act on behalf of the child. This painstaking care before an adoption, though frustrating for adoptive parents, is essential if mistakes are to be avoided. However, this period of waiting means that a baby will be at least four and a half months old before the adoptive parents can be absolutely sure that the baby will not be taken away from them. Once the adoption process is complete, the adopted child is, to all intents and purposes, in exactly the same position as a natural child. A more detailed description of the adoption process and a complete list of all the British adoption agencies is given in a booklet, 'A Brief Guide for Prospective Adopters', obtainable from the British Agencies for Adoption and Fostering (address is given at the end of the book).

The number of babies available for adoption has reduced considerably in recent years. This is partly due to the increased availability of contraception, partly to the more liberal 1967 Abortion Act, and partly because more single mothers are deciding to keep their babies. Single parent families are now relatively common and today it is much more socially acceptable for a single woman to keep her baby. Some improvement in job opportunities for women, and increased welfare provision, also mean that keeping her baby is now more of a practical proposition from the financial point of view than it used to be. An infertile couple who are longing for a child will no doubt be able to appreciate just how heartbreaking it must be for a mother to give up her baby once it is born. If she can possibly manage to keep and support the child herself, it is not surprising that she should do so.

All this means that it is now comparatively rare for a new-born baby to be available for adoption. Waiting lists of hopeful parents are often very long, and in some cases over-subscribed lists have been closed altogether. This does not mean, however, that adoption need necessarily be out of the question; adoption agencies often arrange adoptions of children who, at one time, would have been harder to place. These are usually older children or babies who are handicapped in some way. There are still many of these children available for adoption, and they are in need of loving parents just as much as if they were new-born babies. But a major problem with adoption of this sort is that the needs of these children do not necessarily coincide with the needs of infertile childless couples. The primary task of adoption agencies is to arrange an adoption which meets the need of the child; the needs of the would-be parents are not their primary concern. But most childless couples do not apply to adopt in order to meet the needs of the parentless child; they do so primarily in order to meet their own need, their need for a baby of their own. It is important for couples to understand this difference if they are to make the right decision about adoption. Some of the infertile couples whom we interviewed had decided against adoption because they felt that particular qualities of understanding and acceptance were needed by adoptive parents which they did not possess. For couples who feel they could meet the needs of an older or handicapped child or perhaps a family group of brothers and sisters, the possibility of adoption is still a realistic, practical alternative to remaining childless.

Recently the possibility of adopting babies from a different country has been raised following publicity about the plight of orphans in other countries. Generally the specialised agencies which have a great deal of experience in placing babies for adoption are reluctant to approve such inter-country adoption. These children can be very disturbed and often experience severe problems in settling down in a strange country in addition to adjusting to life within a new family. These official agencies often feel that assistance to improve the quality of child-care in the child's own country would be more advantageous to the children concerned. Very careful enquiries should be made and much thought should be given to the subject before any attempt to adopt a baby from overseas is made.

In-vitro fertilisation

In-vitro fertilisation (IVF) is the mixing of eggs and sperm in a dish in the laboratory to allow fertilisation to occur. It is a complicated and demanding procedure and involves several stages. The woman is treated with drugs which stimulate the development of several eggs within the ovary at one time. The development of these eggs is closely monitored and at the appropriate time they are collected. This is usually done under general anaesthetic. The eggs are prepared and carefully mixed with the prepared sperm of the male partner and placed in an incubator to allow fertilisation to occur. If fertilisation is successful, up to three fertilised eggs are replaced into the woman's uterus using a fine, flexible polythene tube which is inserted through the neck of the womb.

IVF is most frequently used for women whose fallopian tubes are blocked or damaged (see Figure 2 in Chapter 5) but new IVF treatments are now becoming available for those couples where the male partner has a low sperm count or poor quality sperm. The object of these new experimental techniques is to bypass the layer of cells (*the zona pellucida*) which forms a kind of shell around the egg. This layer of cells can prevent sperm which have poor motility or morphology from penetrating and fertilising an egg. In one technique a small hole is made in the zona pellucida which eases the way for the sperm to swim through the hole. Another technique uses a sharp microscopic needle through which the sperm is injected into the egg. These methods are, of course, of no help where the male partner produces no sperm. While it is not a treatment for azoospermia, it is a possibility where oligospermia is present.

All IVF techniques are to some extent experimental, are relatively expensive and the failure rates are high. Success rates vary from centre to centre but overall about nine couples in ten fail to be successful in attempting to have a baby this way. The results of IVF treatment undertaken because of male subfertility tend to be even more disappointing. A decision to undergo IVF needs very careful thought. Several books are available which describe IVF treatment in greater detail and some of these are listed at the end of this book.

Insemination

This is a procedure whereby semen is placed in the woman's vagina by means other than sexual intercourse. Semen is collected by masturbation, placed in a container and then stored by deep-freezing in liquid nitrogen until it is required for use. The semen is placed deep into the vagina near the cervix, or sometimes directly into the cervical canal, by means of a simple narrow plastic tube. (See Figure 2)

The technique of insemination is occasionally used to inseminate a wife with her husband's semen; this is known as artificial insemination by husband (AIH). This procedure was once common but nowadays it is rarely offered. This is because research has shown that introducing the semen into the vagina artificially does not increase its effectiveness. However AIH is sometimes used where there is a physical failure to deliver fertile semen high into the vagina during sexual intercourse. This failure may be because of injury or a malformation of the penis, or because of impotence, or because of vaginal spasm which does not allow the erect penis to penetrate the vagina properly. In such cases a technique that delivers the husband's sperm to the cervix of his wife may have some success in bringing about a pregnancy.

Where the male partner's semen has no fertilising power, semen donated by someone other than the partner can be used. This procedure is called donor insemination (DI). The insemination procedure is the same as for AIH, but the semen is provided by a fertile man who is unknown and unrelated to either partner seeking help. DI is the most common means of establishing a pregnancy through the use of one of the modern infertility treatments collectively described as 'assisted conception' techniques. The remainder of this book is devoted to a detailed consideration of the advantages and disadvantages of using DI as a means of overcoming childlessness.

3

Donor Insemination

Reasons for donor insemination

The majority of couples who undertake DI do so because the male partner is suffering from some degree of subfertility or infertility. As explained in earlier chapters the man, for a variety of reasons, may be unable to produce any sperm, produces insufficient sperm or produces sperm or semen which is abnormal in some way. Any of these problems can make it impossible for fertilisation to occur. But male infertility is not the only reason why DI may be offered.

Sometimes the male partner may suffer from, or be known to carry, an hereditary genetic disorder. Every cell in our bodies carries a kind of blueprint or code which determines our individual make-up and structure. This code or blueprint is contained in the genes. When a baby is conceived the genes from the man and the woman (contained in the sperm and the egg) are rearranged and combined. Whilst each new baby is a unique individual because the genes have been 'shuffled' into his or her own unique code, the basic genetic material is passed on from the parents. Sometimes there is a mistake or abnormality in the genetic code passed on by one of the parents which results in the child being born with a particular disease. A well-known example of this is haemophilia. The statistical odds of passing on a particular genetic disorder which a parent is known to possess can be calculated and it is now possible to receive information from a genetic counsellor about this likelihood. Such information can leave couples with a cruel dilemma. If they conceive they might be fortunate and have a normal baby, but they must take into consideration the strong possibility that the baby will be affected.

Although couples who are carrying a genetic disorder may not have a problem of infertility they share many of the unpleasant emotions which infertile couples experience; complex and disturbing feelings associated with a sense of inadequacy, guilt and self-blame. If the couple are unaware that they are liable to pass on a genetic disorder, the news can be devastating when a baby is found to be affected. One woman whose first baby had inherited a genetic disorder explained:

> It didn't sink in, did it? I know when the doctor told us, he said, 'It's genetic'—and we made no reaction. And he said 'Do you understand what I'm saying?' And we said 'Oh, yes.' We knew what he meant but it took a long time I think before it really sank in exactly what it *did* mean. I don't think it ever does. The fact that we can have children, but it's such a risk. I think *we'd* survive if we had another child and it died, but I don't think I could put a child through it again.

Her husband added:

> It was a very difficult decision to make whether we took a chance and had our own child or . . . it was very difficult. I don't think we were left with too many choices because we had to face the possibility of the same thing happening again and it was just unthinkable.

In the same way as infertile couples, couples known to be carrying a genetic disorder of some sort also need time to work through their feelings of grief and distress before they can reach appropriate decisions about DI. It is in such situations that the help of a skilled independent counsellor can prove invaluable. Although this book is written mainly with infertile couples in mind, much of the information will also be useful in helping to identify and discuss the uncertainties of couples who might be considering DI because of a genetic disorder being carried by one or both partners.

Another reason for childlessness may be a blood group incompatibility between the potential parents. A substance known as the *Rhesus factor* may be absent from the woman's blood, but present in her partner's blood. If a baby which they conceive inherits this Rhesus factor from its father, a reaction occurs in the mother's blood; antibodies are produced which may destroy the baby's blood cells during the baby's development in the uterus. Often the first baby is not badly affected, but subsequent babies may be affected so severely that they do not survive. Fortunately this condition is now much more rare than it was because it is now possible to treat the mother in order to prevent antibodies forming.

An increasingly common reason for couples to consider DI as a way of having children is when the male partner is sterile because of a previous vasectomy operation. The incidence of divorce is increasing and some marriages break up at a relatively late stage after a couple have completed their family and have decided on vasectomy as a permanent form of contraception. Sometimes divorce or separation is followed by the forming of a new partnership. If the new couple then wish to have children of their own they will be unable to do so because the male partner has been sterilised. An operation to reverse vasectomy is sometimes possible but the results are often disappointing. Even if the delivery of the sperm can be restored the fertilising capacity of the semen does not always return. In such cases DI is an option which is often considered.

The development of donor insemination

DI is technically a simple procedure; indeed, DI has been practiced by some couples themselves on a do-it-yourself basis, but the majority of DI treatments are carried out under the supervision of medically qualified practitioners. Semen from a fertile male donor is placed in the reproductive tract of the woman who wishes to conceive using a narrow plastic tube; the procedure is completely painless. This insemination must be carried out at the fertile time in the woman's menstrual cycle, when a mature egg or ovum is released from the surface of the ovary. This release of an ovum is known as ovulation and usually occurs about mid-way between menstrual periods. The semen is sometimes deposited deep in the vagina near the cervix but more usually directly into the entrance of the cervical canal.

Until about a decade ago freshly collected semen was frequently used but since the onset of the AIDS epidemic all semen must be deep frozen and stored in liquid nitrogen for a quarantine period. This period is determined by regulations and is currently six months. This length of time is required to ensure that HIV infection cannot be spread by using semen from infected donors. When needed for use the semen is carefully thawed. Insemination must be accurately timed to take place during the fertile period of a woman's monthly cycle if it is to be successful. The donor remains anonymous and great care is taken to make sure that the donor and the recipient woman do not meet.

DI did not become available in Britain until the late 1930s, when advancing medical knowledge showed that among a considerable number of childless couples it was the male who was the infertile partner. A small group of gynaecologists began to use the technique, but their activities were unknown to the general public until the first report of their work was published in the *British Medical Journal* in 1945. This report provoked a considerable amount of discussion, both in parliament and in the press, and the Archbishop of Canterbury instituted a commission of inquiry which, among other comments, recommended in 1948 that the provision of DI should be made a criminal offence. Following further debate the government appointed an interdepartmental committee, under the chairmanship of Lord Feversham, to make recommendations about the practice of DI. This committee also concluded that DI was undesirable and not to be encouraged, but they feared that if it were made a criminal offence it would merely be driven underground and into the hands of unqualified practitioners. However, the committee felt that as the number of couples seeking DI was small, and the practice was being carried out discreetly by private, medically qualified practitioners, it was probably best left unregulated.

Despite this discouraging start DI continued to be practised and, as infertile couples became more aware of this possible solution to their problems, the demand for DI steadily increased. By 1970 the British Medical Association was receiving sufficiently large numbers of enquiries about DI for them to appoint their own panel of enquiry to look into the whole subject. This committee reported more favourably and recommended, in 1973, that DI should be made available within the National Health Service. Following the development of IVF techniques and the birth of the first test-tube baby in 1978 there was a call for some sort of regulation of the new reproductive technologies and a committee of enquiry under the chairmanship of Lady Warnock was set up. The provision of DI was included in the committee's terms of reference. The report of this committee was published in 1984 and recommended that a licensing authority should be set up to regulate research and the provision of infertility treatments which involved external fertilisation, or the donation of human eggs or sperm. Their recommendations were broadly accepted and were incorporated in the Human Fertilisation and Embryology Act 1990.

Although DI is, from the medical or technical standpoint, a relatively simple procedure, the personal and social implications of the procedure are complex. DI is not a medical treatment in the usual sense; the woman who is being treated is herself quite fit, and the infertility of her partner is not usually being treated at all. It is only if the man and woman are thought of together as a co-operating unit—that is, a couple—that the procedure makes any sense.

Personal and social issues surrounding donor insemination

When a couple marry or decide to set up home together they enter into certain commitments in relation to each other. Each will normally feel they are under certain obligations towards their partner. Each will also feel that they have certain rights within the marriage or relationship and will have expectations about the behaviour of their partner towards them. One clear expectation in our society is that a man and woman living together will have a sexual relationship with his/her spouse, and each expects their partner not to have a sexual relationship with anyone else. Of course these expectations about sexual relationships are not always fulfilled and 'affairs' do sometimes happen, but such an occurrence often leads to a breakdown of that marriage or relationship. Although some people assert that the influence of marriage in our society is becoming weaker, DI illustrates in quite a striking way the strength of the expectation that sexual relationships within marriage must be exclusive. The very fact that those childless couples where the male partner is infertile choose to undergo the inconvenience, stress, embarrassment and financial strain of an impersonal clinical procedure such as DI, rather than achieve a pregnancy by personal sexual intercourse with another man, is clear evidence of this. Looked at this way, DI is dealing with a personal need (the desire for a child of one's own) in a socially acceptable way. It is not medical treatment of the usual kind because a cure of the man's infertility is not being provided. DI resolves childlessness but not infertility. However, DI fulfils a personal need, that of obtaining a child whilst at the same time maintaining an exclusive sexual relationship with one's partner. Because the insemination is impersonal and 'artificial', the exclusive physical sexual relationship of the couple is maintained.

If DI is meeting a personal need and not a medical need, why then is the medical profession so deeply involved in its provision? Part of this involvement comes about because the initial investigation of infertility is most definitely a medical issue. However, other purely medical justifications are hard to find. Of course the fertile time of the woman's monthly cycle must be determined, and the genetic father of the child—the donor—must be recruited, but medical expertise is not strictly necessary for this. The main reason for the involvement of the medical profession in DI treatment provision appears, again, to be more social than medical. The doctor acts as an 'honest broker', mediating between the couple and a suitable donor. The professional standing of the doctor tends to legitimise the procedure and gives it respectability, and both the donor and the couple are reassured and given added confidence that their involvement in the DI procedure will be handled responsibly.

Most couples are well aware that DI is more than a medical matter and that it has serious implications for their own and other family relationships. While DI maintains an exclusive sexual relationship it does not maintain an exclusive reproductive relationship; it does not enable a man to reproduce. Though the male partner will become the father of any child that is born following DI, he is not the *genetic* father, the procreator of that child. This is a difficult situation for most men to face. Until fairly recently couples were encouraged to believe there was no need for anyone to know that the child conceived by DI had a different genetic father, and that it was best if they tried to forget about the donor's involvement. But maintaining such a secret carries with it a psychological price, and pretending that something has never happened is rarely a satisfactory way of resolving a situation. Most people who have studied the personal implications of DI now believe that the energy spent in denying infertility and hiding DI is better spent in trying to understand and accept the situation as it really is. To want to keep DI secret implies that there is something shameful about infertility and DI. This is not so, and there is no reason why couples who have a DI child should not feel as proud of their parenthood as any other couple. Although parenthood is achieved in a different way, it is keenly sought and usually achieved at considerable emotional cost. Among the couples we interviewed who have DI children, many had told friends and relatives and all were glad that they had done so. Their confidants had been understanding and had generally offered wholehearted support and encouragement. It is vitally important that couples who are considering DI as a solution to their childlessness should be aware of, and should discuss fully with each other, the social implications of the procedure for themselves and their families.

Comparison of donor insemination with adoption

When making the decision about whether or not to seek DI, most couples also consider adoption as an alternative means of dealing with their childlessness. The couples we interviewed saw many differences between adoption and DI and almost all expressed the view that DI had advantages over adoption. Perhaps the most commonly expressed opinion was that the child was more 'theirs' because it was part of at least one of them. DI also made it possible for a woman to *bear* a child, whereas adoption only permitted her to *rear* a child born to another woman; adoption would not give her the opportunity of experiencing pregnancy and childbirth. Couples felt that the joint experience of pregnancy and childbirth which DI had made possible (most husbands or partners were present at the birth) gave them a closer and stronger bond with their child. While a genetic link was present with only one of them, the couple had, together, experienced the detailed planning of the child's birth. The DI parents were aware that if they had adopted a child they would have been taking over responsibility for a child who already existed and who had originated outside their own relationship; but their DI child resulted directly from a decision made by themselves and would never have been born otherwise. One couple explained: 'We both desperately wanted a child that was *ours* right from the very start. Part of *our* unit. We didn't want somebody just to come and knock at the door and say, 'Right, we've got a baby for you.'' Another man explained the difference between DI and adoption very concisely: 'DI is the act of creation, whereas adoption is a sort of accommodation.'

4

The Donor Insemination Service

How is the provision of donor insemination regulated?

The provision of DI is controlled and regulated by the legislation contained in the Human Fertilisation and Embryology Act (1990). This Act required the setting up of an independent Human Fertilisation and Embryology Authority to control and licence centres offering treatment using donated sperm or eggs, or treatment involving the creation of human embryos outside the body. The storage of human sperm, eggs or embryos and the conduct of research is also controlled. The Act requires that in any decision about the provision of a regulated treatment, account must be taken of the welfare of any child who may be born as a result of treatment (including the need of that child for a father) and of any other children who may be affected by the birth. In addition, donors and recipients of donated eggs or sperm must be provided with relevant information and be given a suitable opportunity to receive proper counselling before giving written consent to their participation in any treatment.

Proper records, including details of the persons donating or receiving sperm (or eggs or embryos) and details of any child born as a result of the regulated treatment, must be maintained by centres and forwarded to the Human Fertilisation and Embryology Authority (HFEA). The HFEA is required to keep a register containing information about donors and about people who are provided with treatment together with details of the outcome of treatment. The purpose of the register is to enable the HFEA to monitor the provision of DI in treatment centres and to provide certain types of information to those who are entitled to make enquiries. A person who is born following DI has a right to receive certain limited information at the age of 18 years (or from 16 years if they are to be married). Before giving this information, the enquirer has to be offered (but does not have to accept) an opportunity to receive 'proper' counselling. No clear description of what is meant by 'proper' counselling is given but it is assumed this would be provided by a trained counsellor who is independent of the team providing the DI treatment. The law prohibits the giving of information which may identify a sperm, egg or embryo donor. An enquirer will be informed if the partner with whom she/he intends to have children might be related (to guard against the possibility of the anonymous donor being a parent of them both) but no identifying information about the donor can be divulged. The HFEA is required to maintain a code of practice which is intended to assist those wishing to provide or use the regulated services. Treatment centres which provide DI must be licensed and operate according to this code of practice drawn up by the Authority. Inspectors of the HFEA visit these centres each year to make certain that the terms of the licence are being adhered to. While infringement of the code does not of itself constitute a criminal offence, the renewal of the required licence to provide a service or undertake research may be refused if the code is not being followed.

Where can donor insemination treatment be obtained?

Private medical practitioners were the pioneers in providing a DI service and the majority of centres providing DI in this country still do so on a private or semi-private fee-paying basis. In 1973 a committee of the

British Medical Association recommended that DI should be made available on the National Health Service as a regular part of the provision of infertility services. A few NHS centres have been set up but the demand for treatment is heavy and so waiting lists at NHS centres are usually very long. In some areas the demand has been so great, and the waiting lists have grown so long, that the consultant in charge has felt it necessary to impose a residence qualification upon new patients, and only couples living within a specified distance of the centre are accepted for treatment. Unfortunately, funds within the NHS are scarce and the priority given to infertility services is not high. Some centres have been set up in NHS teaching hospitals in co-operation with university medical school departments, but because NHS funds are not available these centres have to charge a fee. The aim of infertility specialists is to have sufficient NHS centres so that no couple needs to travel more than 40 miles to reach a centre, and the maximum time spent on a waiting list should be no longer than six months. This aim has yet to be achieved and organisations set up to promote the interests of infertile couples are working hard to draw attention to the need for a higher priority to be given to the provision of infertility services.

Couples who wish to be referred for DI should first approach their own general practitioner; he or she normally will be able to provide information about where to find the nearest NHS (or private) centre offering a service. More likely, a referral will be made to a gynaecology or infertility clinic for further investigation or treatment. If there is no NHS centre providing DI nearby, or if the waiting list is very long, couples may wish to consider attending a private centre. A list of such centres is available to family doctors from the Royal College of Obstetricians & Gynaecologists or from the Human Fertilisation and Embryology Authority. Sometimes family doctors leave it to their patients to take the initiative in asking about DI. DI is a serious and controversial step and not one to be undertaken lightly. It is therefore an added safeguard if doctors adopt a rather cautious attitude. But sometimes a doctor may have moral or religious scruples about DI which are not shared by the couple, and as a result may be reluctant to refer a patient. One enquirer said to us:

> My doctor tended to put me off. He was far more keen on us going for adoption. I had to fight. I had to be very adamant and say, 'I want to go to her [the DI specialist]. Will you please refer me?'—and he did.

There are various organisations which can also be approached to give local information about the provision of DI. Contrary to popular belief, the Family Planning Association is not solely interested in preventing unwanted births, but also offers help and advice in planning the birth of wanted children. The telephone number of the nearest FPA information centre will be in the local telephone directory. 'Issue', a national association of childless couples, is also able to offer information about DI and to give details of its provision. 'Issue' produces information leaflets and a quarterly newsletter, and there are local groups in many areas where couples can meet each other and discuss problems and provide mutual support. Another organisation called 'Child' also offers help and information to infertile couples and has local area groups where couples can meet and share their problems and ideas. (Addresses and telephone numbers for these organisations are given at the end of the book.)

What factors should be taken into account when choosing a treatment centre?

The quality of the medical treatment (if not the plush surroundings) available in NHS centres is of a standard which will equal, and may well surpass, that available in private centres. Several NHS centres situated in different parts of the country are set up within university teaching hospitals and are headed by consultants who are at the forefront of research and development in infertility treatments. Under the new market system of purchasers and providers within the NHS, fundholding family doctors may be able to refer some patients to specialist NHS clinics outside their immediate area. However, in general the NHS is short of funds and infertility treatments are not given a high priority. Such services are therefore considerably overstretched. Many patients find the waiting list for treatment is long and there may be long delays between appointments. Some couples, particularly older couples who fear time might be running out for them, find this delay very frustrating and prefer to seek treatment at a private centre where the waiting time is usually much shorter.

A couple's family doctor may be able to recommend a private centre, but there is nothing to prevent couples from making their own enquiries. A family doctor is unlikely to object if asked to refer a couple to a treatment centre of their own choice, and may be able to provide a list of local addresses to choose from. It is advisable not to rush this choice of centre; there is a financial cost for treatment and success is not guaranteed. Couples should identify 3 or 4 centres which can be reached fairly easily and then telephone them for information about their facilities. Any information leaflets which the centres provide should be obtained in advance of any treatment and the facilities being offered at each of the centres should be compared. Answers to the following questions might be used as a guide:

How much does treatment cost and what is included in this cost?

How frequently is attendance at the centre required?

If success is not immediate for how long is treatment available?

What is the rate of success reported by the centre?

What sort of treatment record is kept?

Will the same doctor or nurse be seen at each visit?

What facilities are there for husbands or partners?

How are donors recruited?
Is an independent counsellor linked to the centre?
Is there a support group?
Is there a complaints procedure if any difficulties arise?

Before finally deciding on a particular centre it is worth making a visit to the centre to see the facilities at first hand and to get the feel of the place. It is important that the couple should feel comfortable in the centre and with the staff, and confident about the quality of the treatment they are likely to receive. Some of the questions listed here are dealt with in more detail in the pages which follow.

How much will donor insemination treatment cost?

The provision of DI is rarely completely free even at NHS centres because NHS funds are not usually available to cover all the costs of providing the service. For example, the expenses which are paid to donors or the laboratory costs of freeze-storing semen may have to be met by the couple.

Costs at a private centre will depend on which centre a couple decide to attend, as fees within the private sector vary quite widely. The initial consultation is usually a lengthy one to allow time for the doctor and the couple to discuss the implications of DI together, and so the fee for this first consultation is often higher than for the subsequent more routine visits. Some centres do not charge a separate fee for each individual consultation, but have one combined total fee which covers a whole period of inseminations, perhaps the first three-month or six-month period. This means that if the couple are fortunate and conception occurs quickly at the first or second visit, they will have paid in advance for visits which they will not make. On the other hand it may be necessary for more than one insemination to be performed in some menstrual cycles and so payment for individual visits may become the more costly system. Sometimes the consultation fee quoted does not cover additional items such as laboratory tests, drugs which may be prescribed, or ultrasound scans and these may be charged separately over and above the basic consultation fee. This can increase the costs of treatment considerably.

Official reports of costs show a wide variation; much depends on what is included in the total package. Couples should expect to pay (at 1993 prices) between £85 and £400 for each treatment cycle. This refers to the cost of treatment provided in one menstrual cycle only; the full cost is calculated by multiplying the cost for each cycle by the number of menstrual cycles in which treatment takes place. As a rough guide it is estimated that there is an average success rate of 50% in achieving a pregnancy within 5 treatment cycles. Depending on the centre where DI treatment is being obtained this will require an average outlay of between £435 and £2000 with an even chance that a pregnancy will be achieved. With total costs in this range it is wise for couples to decide, in advance of starting treatment, how much they are willing to spend. Once treatment has started it is sometimes very difficult to come to a decision to stop, with the danger that costs can rise to an unintended level. It is important when comparing the costs charged by different centres to ensure that like is being compared with like. Our experience of visiting centres suggests that the high prices charged at some centres are not necessarily equated with a greater success rate in achieving a pregnancy and the wide variation in costs is not necessarily reflected in the quality of the service provided.

The various private medical insurance associations have different policies regarding DI, but generally infertility treatment is not covered by private medical insurance. Some insurers provide cover for infertility investigations but insurance cover must pre-date the diagnosis of infertility before associations will accept liability. Couples who have private health insurance should check carefully the extent of their cover before embarking on treatment.

Couples should also realise that medical fees are not the only costs involved in having DI. Many couples have to travel long distances to DI clinics, and travelling expenses may add considerably to the overall bill and may even exceed medical costs. Time taken off work in order to attend for regular inseminations may also lead to loss of earnings and so further add to the costs of DI.

Can donor insemination treatment be obtained outside licensed centres?

It is known that some women have arranged DI for themselves without involving the medical profession. The process of insemination itself is very simple, and it is possible for a woman to inseminate herself using donated semen on a 'do-it yourself' basis. Accurate timing of the insemination is the most difficult part of treatment. However because the woman can perform the insemination herself more frequently than a visit to a treatment centre often permits, accurate prediction of the time of ovulation is not so necessary. The women who do this are often single women who wish to have their own child but who do not wish to enter into a long-term relationship with a man. A friend (or perhaps a friend of a friend) is asked to act as an intermediary in finding a fertile man who is willing to donate semen. So long as this is not done as a commercial transaction it is not illegal.

There are, however, problems which can be encountered in this course of action. Perhaps the most obvious is the possibility of the transmission of HIV infection; where DI takes place outside an officially recognised centre there is no medical screening of donors. Child maintenance payments may also be required from the donor. When DI is provided in licensed centres the anonymous donor has no financial or legal obligations towards any child born as a result of his donation. In 'unofficial' DI the donor is legally recognised as the father and, as such, is held responsible for the financial support of any child who may be born as a result of his semen donation; this support would be enforced through the payment of child maintenance contributions.

Occasionally a woman, or a couple, may also consider seeking direct help from a donor who is known to them, perhaps a relative or a close friend. This could create problems in addition to those described above, resulting from the complexity of conflicting relationships which could arise as the child grows up. While DI might be simple in terms of its technology, the social and psychological effects of its use can be exceedingly complex. It is important to ensure that the interests of all those taking part in DI and above all the resulting child, are carefully considered. These interests are most effectively protected if the provision of DI treatment is properly regulated.

Is is possible to have regulated donor insemination treatment at home?

Regulated DI treatment normally must be provided only in treatment centres licensed and inspected by the HFEA. However, in exceptional circumstances where a woman is suffering from some disability which prevents her attending a centre (for example, agoraphobia) arrangements can be made to treat her at home. If necessary, enquiries about this should be made at a local treatment centre.

How common is donor insemination?

Starting in the early 1940s in this country DI was provided for a relatively small number of couples. It was not until the 1970s that the demand for DI dramatically increased. Until this time most infertile couples had traditionally looked to adoption to solve their problem of childlessness. During the 1970s, however, the number of babies available for adoption was greatly reduced with the result that the likelihood of being offered a baby to adopt was not a realistic one for most couples. This meant that infertile couples, at least those couples where the woman was fertile and able to bear a child, began to look to DI as a solution to their childlessness. Publicity about the advances in external fertilisation techniques (*in-vitro* fertilisation) also gave added publicity to the availability of DI. This meant that many more couples became aware of the possibility of having DI to alleviate their childlessness and this too increased the demand for DI services.

At the present time there are no figures available which give accurate details of the numbers of DI births each year. This will change when the records of the Human Fertilisation and Embryology Authority become available following the legal requirement that the outcome of DI treatment is recorded. While it is known that such births number several thousand each year, precise numbers have been difficult to determine because DI children are registered in the same way as naturally conceived children. However, it is possible for those involved in DI provision to make a reasonable guess about the figures: during the 1980s it was estimated that about 2,000 children were born in Britain each year as a result of DI. (It is thought that in the United States of America about 15,000 such babies are born annually.) There are also well-established and widespread DI services in Canada, Denmark, Norway, France, Belgium, Holland, Sweden, Japan, New Zealand and Australia in addition to those in the USA and the UK. One doctor has suggested that in a community where DI provision exists, DI births will account for only 1 or 2 births in every 1,000 births in that community. However, as knowledge of the availability of DI increases, it is likely that the demand for DI will also increase. An experienced practitioner writing in a recent issue of an international medical journal estimated that DI offers the only means of achieving a pregnancy for about one-quarter of all infertile couples. With infertility being experienced by about 10% of all couples in the UK, the writer considers it likely that the use of DI will continue to increase, and in contrast to the earlier estimate, he suggests that the procedure could eventually be responsible for up to 2 in every 100 babies being born.

Is donor insemination an accepted procedure?

Whilst DI is an accepted procedure in the medical sense, it would be untrue to pretend that the procedure is completely accepted in the social sense. Many religious denominations have made statements rejecting DI. Pope Pius XII condemned the practice in 1951 and this remains the teaching of the Roman Catholic Church. The Archbishop of Canterbury in 1948 argued that the practice of DI should be made illegal and a criminal offence. A committee of the Church of England which reported in 1960 disagreed with the archbishop, but nevertheless considered such treatment to be 'undesirable and immoral'. Moral and religious attitudes have, of course, changed over the years and many people who are practising members of religious denominations no longer feel bound by the official pronouncements of their church leaders. Such people often feel they must obey their own conscience, taking wider ethical issues into account. This attitude appears to be similar to that relating to the use of contraceptives in order to control excess fertility. For example, there are numbers of practising Roman Catholics who cannot accept their church's teaching on contraception and who use forbidden methods of birth control with a clear conscience. The attitudes of church leaders have also changed and many no longer generally condemn the practice of DI, preferring to consider each case on its merits and to take into account the individual circumstances. In response to consultations during the drafting of the 1990 Human Fertilisation and Embryology Act, the Protestant churches raised some concerns about the procedure. They were concerned about the effect DI might have on family relationships, and on the consequences for the donor and his present or future family. They also expressed disquiet that at that time there was much secrecy surrounding DI. The child was usually deceived into believing that he or she was the natural child of the husband, and close relatives, particularly grandparents, were often similarly deceived. They were also concerned that there was no legal framework for the correct birth registration of children born following DI, and that unlike adopted children they had no right of access to the identity of their biological parent.

Of course many couples may argue that they do not belong to any church and so are unaffected by the comments of religious bodies. However, all these points are legitimate areas of concern and not solely about religious opinions or beliefs, but are concerns shared by many other people. The content of the 1990 Act addressed many (but not all) of these concerns, and there is little doubt that the new legislative control over the procedure has brought with it a greater degree of formal acceptance of DI. There is now a legal framework for the registration of the birth of children following treatment and many of the ethical and social issues which caused concern have been addressed in the Act. But it must still be acknowledged that the procedure remains controversial and is not universally accepted. The legislation encourages a greater degree of openness in the provision of DI. If this comes about it is to be expected that as society in general becomes better informed about DI, and aware of the hard choices which infertile couples must make, there will be the opportunity for the development of a more tolerant and understanding public attitude to this means of achieving a family.

Can anyone have donor insemination treatment?

It is important to understand at the outset that DI is appropriate only when the woman herself is fertile; DI offers no solution to female infertility. If there is any reason to doubt a woman's fertility, a doctor may wish to carry out tests to make certain that she is capable of bearing children before DI is commenced. There is no formal upper age limit beyond which couples are not accepted for treatment, however it is generally accepted that in most women the level of fertility begins to decline normally after the age of about 35 years. Some centres, particularly those which have a very long waiting list, may feel that it is unfair to the younger people on the waiting list to keep them waiting while the centre treats older women, perhaps over the age of 40 years, who have a reduced likelihood of achieving a pregnancy because of their age. This is not to say that all women over the age of 40 are unlikely to become pregnant but a recognition that among these older women natural fertility is reduced.

There is no formal selection or assessment of couples for DI comparable with the way that prospective adoptive parents are chosen. However the legislation regulating the provision of DI requires that account must be taken of the welfare of any child who may be born as a result of treatment (including the need of that child for a father) and of any other children who may be affected by the birth. This means that when deciding whether or not to provide treatment the treatment team has a legal responsibility to consider not just the wishes of the couple who are seeking help but also the needs of any child who may be born as result of DI treatment. The code of practice which provides guidance to centres on how to provide a DI service suggests that the decision whether or not to provide DI treatment should be based on such factors as:

- the ages and medical histories of the couple;
- the commitment of each of them to bringing up a child conceived by DI;
- the effect of a new baby on any existing child of the family;
- a child's potential need to know about his or her origins and whether or not the prospective parents are prepared for the questions which may arise while the child is growing up;
- the possible attitudes of other members of the family towards the child;
- any possibility of a dispute about legal fatherhood.

The centre is also advised to make enquiries of the couple's family doctor about these matters because the doctor will probably have known the couple over a period of time and is likely to be in a better position to offer relevant advice. The centre must obtain the consent of the couple before attempting to make any contact with the family doctor and the couple has the right to refuse permission. However, a refusal to give consent would be taken into account in any decision about whether or not treatment will be offered. This decision is the responsibility of the doctor in charge of treatment but the official code of practice suggests that before reaching this decision, he/she should be sensitive to the views of the other members of the treatment team. In this way care is taken to ensure that each application for DI treatment is considered carefully and in the absence of individual preferences or prejudices.

Up to this point we have assumed that it will be a couple seeking treatment but this is not always so. Single women also occasionally seek DI treatment and there are no legal grounds for refusing to provide this treatment simply because a woman is unmarried or is not accompanied by a male partner. However, the situation is not as straightforward as this statement might suggest. While the Human Fertilisation and Embryology Act does not refer to marriage as a condition for receiving DI treatment it does require centres only to provide DI (and other regulated treatments) after account has been taken of any potential child's need for a father.

Single parent families are becoming much more common and more accepted, and this is used as an argument to support the practice of providing DI for single women. Whilst some may argue that the choice of whether or not to seek DI treatment should be the woman's alone, the child to be born is also affected by this choice. The law requires that the welfare of the child is taken into account and this sometimes means that the decision whether or not to provide treatment can be very difficult for the treatment team.

In the case of adoption, selection of couples is undertaken because the needs and rights of a child already born have to be safeguarded. If adoption societies are to fulfil their responsibility to the child, they have a duty to do all they can to ensure that the couple to whom they entrust the child will make good parents. It is as if the rest of society has taken some responsibility for the child. Such responsibility is covered by carefully designed rules which are strictly observed. The essential difference between babies born as a result of a private act between consenting adults and the giving of a baby by adoption is that, in the case of adoption, people other than the biological parents are involved. In the case of accepting a woman for DI treatment there is as yet no child, but the same argument applies. People other than the parents are involved in the creation of the child. Of course, we all know that there are no restrictions placed upon becoming 'natural' parents (provided these parents conform to the law governing the age of the potential mother and those forbidding incest). Natural parents may even behave irresponsibly or cruelly towards their children, but no one suggests they should be selected or assessed in some way before being allowed to have a child. Many of the couples we have talked with often use this argument as a reason for opposing any routine selection procedure for DI couples. One woman expressed it this way:

> Couples who are fertile can have babies anyway—it's just something that happens whether they are unsuitable parents or highly suitable. So I think everybody should be given the opportunity if they want it.

This feeling is very understandable, but it fails to take account of the fact that DI couples are not just going ahead on their own. They are involving other people to implement their decision, in this case the semen donor and the treatment team of nurses, doctors, counsellors, laboratory technicians and other support staff. These people have professional responsibilities as well as a legal duty not to engage in something they suspect might cause harm to an individual, even if that individual has yet to be born. This means that occasionally a doctor may feel that it is inappropriate for his/her team to provide DI for a particular couple.

The couples we interviewed, whilst in the main being against a formal selection or rejection process, were also aware that DI would not be the right answer for every childless couple. One man said: 'A couple could go and have that done and then the husband either rejects the child, or the wife rejects the husband because he is not the father of that child.' Another woman said:

> I don't think the situation would work where perhaps a woman went [to the clinic], and perhaps her husband didn't want children like this, but she's made up her mind she's going to have children one way or another. Because unless you both want a child, and a child that way, then no way would it work.

It is very important that a couple give full consideration to their decision about whether or not to seek DI treatment. It is essential for them to discuss it together at length and for them to listen to, and respect, each other's point of view. It is now a requirement that all treatment centres should provide an opportunity to discuss the implications of DI treatment with a skilled counsellor. This facility also includes the provision of a place where discussion can take place in private and where interruption is unlikely. It is our view that time spent with a counsellor is well worth while and can be extremely beneficial both in the short term and in the longer term. The main task of the counsellor is to provide an opportunity for the couple to examine the implications of DI treatment for themselves, their immediate families and for the child yet to be born and to examine their own feelings in an informed and non-judgemental way. Couples already experiencing some stress because of their infertility and who may be preoccupied with their own needs may find it difficult to consider the welfare of a child, especially one not yet conceived. It may be particularly difficult for the potential parent to accept that a child's needs and welfare might not always be consistent with their own desires. By taking up the opportunity to participate in counselling a couple is more likely to come to a well-founded, informed decision about DI treatment. In the few cases where DI treatment is inadvisable, it is better if the couple discover this for themselves.

5

Undergoing Donor Insemination Treatment

What does donor insemination treatment entail?

As we have already pointed out, DI is only appropriate when the woman is herself fertile and able to conceive a child. This means that at some centres treatment will not commence until tests and investigations of the woman's fertility have been carried out and these have shown that conception and pregnancy are possible. The treatment team at other centres may be willing to presume fertility is present without the need for these tests provided there is evidence of good general health, there are no obvious gynaecological problems, and that menstrual periods are normal and regular. In such cases, tests and investigations of fertility are only likely to take place if there is a failure to conceive during the first few months of DI treatment.

The timing of the insemination appointments is vital: they have to coincide with the fertile period of the woman's menstrual cycle if a successful conception is to be achieved. The fertile days of the menstrual cycle are those when the ovum or egg is ripening and being released from the surface of the ovary to begin its journey down the fallopian tube towards the uterus or womb. The release of the egg from the surface of the ovary is known as *ovulation*, and this usually takes place about mid-way between the periods of menstrual bleeding. The egg can only survive for a short while after ovulation unless it is

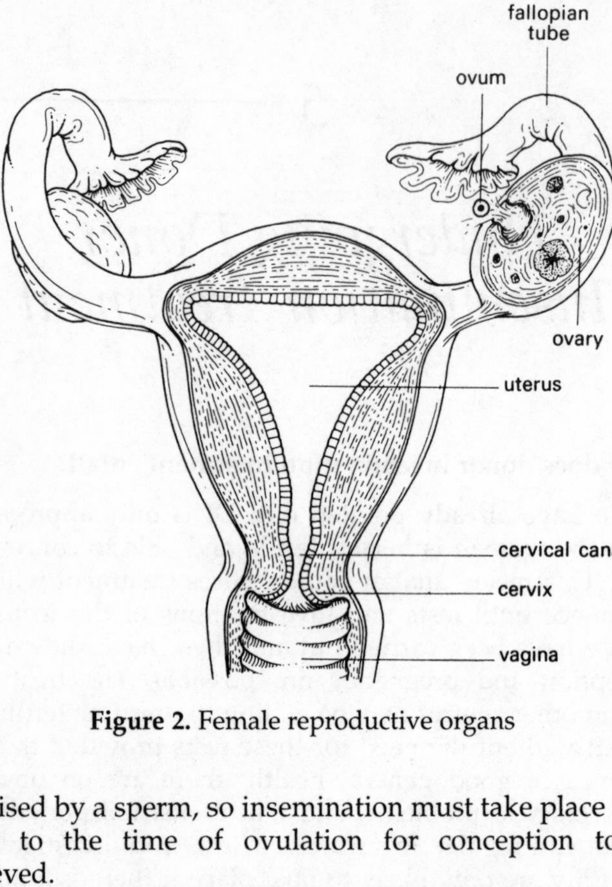

Figure 2. Female reproductive organs

fertilised by a sperm, so insemination must take place very close to the time of ovulation for conception to be achieved.

The time of ovulation must therefore be pinpointed with considerable accuracy if an insemination is to be successful. This is harder than is often supposed; it is not simply a matter of counting on a certain number of days from the start of the previous menstrual period, because the date of ovulation is related to the *next* period and not the one just experienced. In a 28-day cycle ovulation usually takes place approximately 14 or 15 days *before* the day the next period commences. If, as is common, the cycle length is not always of 28 days, the calculation of ovulation by timing it from the last menstrual period becomes a matter of guesswork and is often inaccurate.

So an attempt has to be made to predict ovulation as accurately as possible by other means. It is the determination of the timing of ovulation which is perhaps the most important element in successful DI treatment.

The most common way in which the timing of ovulation is predicted is by taking the temperature of the body every day and noting when a change in temperature, which is known to be related to ovulation, first takes place. This temperature has to be taken when the body is resting (this is known as the basal body temperature) and at the same time each day, first thing each morning before getting out of bed. When ovulation occurs the basal body temperature rises by about 0.2°C from its previous level and stays at this higher level until just before the next menstrual period when it falls back to its original level. The temperature rise, provided it is maintained over several days, indicates that ovulation has taken place for that cycle. As 0.2°C is a fairly small temperature change to detect, the temperature must be taken carefully and conscientiously at the same time every day using a special fertility thermometer. Sometimes the DI treatment specialist may ask that body temperature is taken for two or three months and the result recorded on a special chart before commencing DI treatment. In this way a woman's pattern of menstruation and ovulation can be determined on an individual basis. This increases the accuracy with which ovulation in the next menstrual cycle can be predicted and this in turn helps the treatment team to plan when a DI appointment is most likely to coincide with the fertile period. It is very possible that women seeking DI treatment will be asked to maintain this temperature record throughout the duration of treatment.

Another way of recognising the fertile period is to note the quality of the mucus which appears at the entrance to the vagina. In the first few days after a menstrual period any mucus which is present at the vaginal opening is usually thick, cloudy and 'sticky' in consistency. As the time of ovulation approaches, the amount of mucus increases and its consistency changes; it becomes clear, slippery and 'stretchy'. Some writers have described this mucus as resembling raw egg-white. This type of mucus aids the movement of sperm towards the fallopian tube. It is in the fallopian tube that the sperm, if successful, will fertilise the ovum which has just been shed from the ovary. If a woman can learn to recognise the change in the quantity and consistency of this mucus it can be a valuable pointer to the onset of ovulation and another aid in timing the insemination appointment accurately.

Thirdly, blood tests or urine tests can be used to measure the levels of various hormones in the woman's body which are known to fluctuate at the time of ovulation. Prediction of ovulation using laboratory tests of this sort is more accurate than the other methods described but their use may involve additional early morning visits to the treatment centre. These are not always easily arranged or feasible if the woman has to travel some distance. Some centres may also offer the use of ultrasound scanning to examine the ovaries to determine if ovulation is about to occur.

These attempts to determine the time of ovulation are all used as aids to reduce, as much as possible, the margin of error in predicting ovulation. Appointments for DI treatment must be flexible and are often made at short notice. The Fertility Committee of the Royal College of Obstetricians and Gynaecologists advises that where possible treatment centres should be open on a daily basis; if this is not possible there should be at least three clinics per week held on alternate days. In some centres women are asked to telephone the clinic in the morning with up-to-date information about temperature or mucus changes, and an appointment may be given for later that day if the changes suggest it would be appropriate. Nevertheless, an accurate prediction of the date of ovulation remains a difficult task, particularly if the menstrual cycle is irregular, and this is one reason why a successful insemination can be elusive.

Most centres have a waiting list and are unable to commence DI immediately a couple is referred to the centre for treatment. Provided the waiting time is not *too* long, this enforced pause can have advantages. It gives a couple time to discuss very thoroughly with each other what their own feelings and views are, and to be quite sure and certain about their decision to go ahead with DI.

The insemination procedure itself is a very simple one. Many centres encourage the husband or male partner to attend the appointment too. The woman lies either on her side or her back, in the same position as that adopted for an internal examination. An instrument known as a speculum is placed in the vagina; this enables the *cervix*, or opening of the womb into the vagina, to be seen clearly. Fertile semen is then placed either around or just inside the cervix, using a narrow polythene tube; the speculum is then removed. The whole procedure is quite painless. Afterwards, the woman is usually asked to lie down for about 20 minutes with her buttocks slightly raised to prevent the semen draining away from the locality of the cervix. The semen must have been deep frozen and kept for a quarantine period of at least six months. It is thawed out just before use. It is fairly common for a trained nurse, working under the supervision of a doctor, to carry out this insemination procedure. Sometimes only one insemination is performed in each menstrual cycle—particularly if the couple live a long way from the centre—but some centres follow a procedure whereby two or more inseminations are provided during each menstrual cycle whenever this is possible. By providing a number of opportunities during each menstrual cycle, the determination of the precise timing of ovulation is less critical and this is likely to be reflected in the rate of success in achieving a pregnancy.

Whilst the procedure is technically very simple, insemination can sometimes be psychologically trying and stressful for the couple concerned. We say this not to put couples off or to discourage them, but because 'to be forewarned is to be forearmed', as the saying goes. This stress mainly comes about because couples are so very keen to get pregnant. When a woman has not conceived

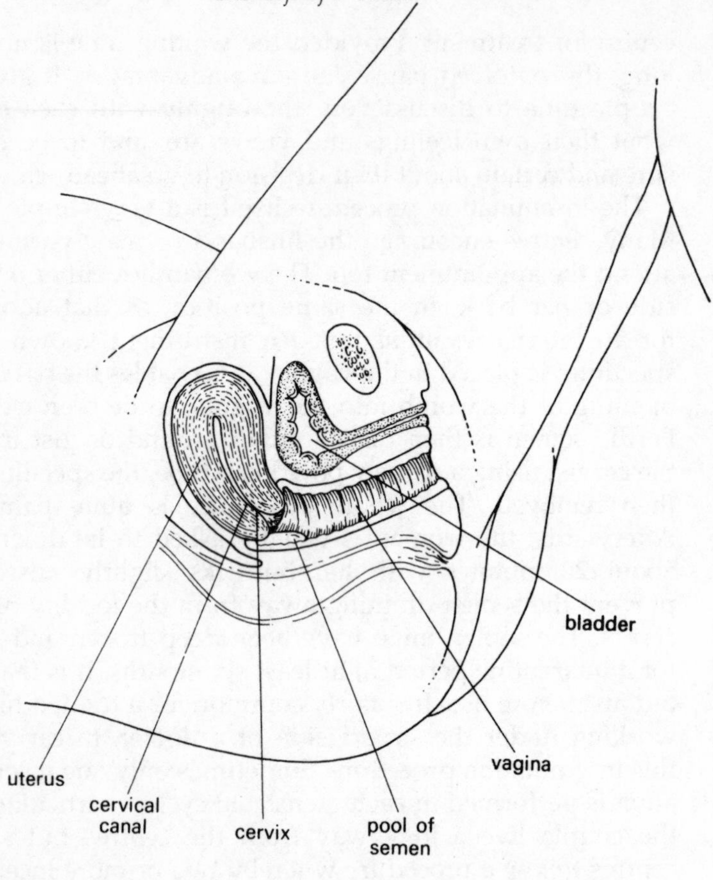

Figure 3. Female reproductive tract after insemination

after an insemination, and her menstrual period arrives again as usual, she can become very disappointed and despondent. One woman expressed the frustration associated with the cyclical pattern of hope followed by despondency in the following way: 'The disappointment when your period starts, it's so intense because for a full two weeks you are hoping, and then you go down so quickly.'

Taking a temperature every day can also increase the strain, because this is a continuous reminder of the longing for a child and the hope that *this time* the treatment will be successful. These feelings are difficult to ignore even for a short time. Another woman recalled her feelings about this:

> One of the most depressing things I find is that you can never, ever put it out of your mind and forget about it, because every morning you have to take your temperature—it's always with you whether you're on holiday, or Christmas, or whatever.

Asking for time off work in order to attend the centre once or twice a month for several months in succession can also sometimes be a source of stress. This stress can be increased if there is also a long, tiring and expensive journey to be undertaken in order to get to the centre.

However, by no means all couples get anxious and stressed, and action can be taken to ease the stress that does occur. The first step is to recognise that stress might (and often does) occur and then to take positive steps to deal with it. It may seem obvious to say so, but it is helpful if the couple seeking treatment have hobbies or leisure pursuits which 'take them out of themselves' for a time; anything that prevents those involved from being *solely* pre-occupied with the business of getting pregnant can be beneficial. Sometimes couples feel hesitant about discussing their infertility problems and their decision to seek DI treatment with their immediate family and with close friends. This has the disadvantage of closing off an escape valve by which some of the frustration and tension can be released. The couples we talked with who have told close friends or relatives about having DI, and about their hopes for a baby, are all very glad that they have done so. Their confidants are reported as being, without exception, understanding and supportive and have proved to be a great strength and comfort in difficult times. One woman said: 'I'm very close to my mother. We talk about it and it makes it a lot easier.' Her husband added: 'You don't want to take all the burden on your own shoulders.' Another couple had looked to close friends for support:

> So we took [friends] into our confidence, and they were very supportive. And we could talk to them about it. I think to have made the decision to keep it totally to ourselves would have made it very difficult, particularly in the anxious times.

Couples are now encouraged to be more open about their infertility problems and their intention to seek DI treatment. By sharing hopes and disappointments with a trusted and supportive relative or friend the inevitable anxieties and uncertainties which accompany DI treatment can be greatly reduced.

Is membership of a patient support group helpful?

It is very common these days for people who are encountering similar difficulties to join together in what are usually called "self-help" groups. These groups offer a valuable opportunity for members to share their experiences and to exchange useful ideas for dealing with problems. Many centres now organise patient support groups which meet at a time and place convenient to the group members. The aim is to provide an opportunity for individuals and couples who are having—or planning to have—DI treatment to meet together in an informal way. Occasionally a speaker might be invited to talk about a relevant topic, and usually the sister in charge of the clinic and the counsellor will be available to attend the group if they are asked. Meeting other people who have similar problems gives couples the chance to see the various ways other people cope. It is also reassuring to know that one's own experiences are not unique, or even unusual.

How successful is donor insemination treatment?

Although success cannot be measured just by physical results, most people take this question to mean 'How likely am I to get pregnant?'. Success rates can be measured in different ways; sometimes the statistics refer to the success rate *per treatment cycle* and sometimes they refer to the rate of success *per couple* who commence treatment. On average 50 to 60 per cent of couples who commence DI achieve a pregnancy. This leaves between a third and a half of couples who do not achieve a pregnancy as a result of DI treatment. Of course, figures vary from centre to centre and some achieve a higher percentage of pregnancies than these figures suggest. This is possibly because some centres are more selective about the couples they accept, and require some evidence that the woman who is to receive donor sperm is likely to be fertile. The partner of an infertile man may also be suffering from some degree of infertility or subfertility herself and so may be unable to conceive on her own account. The age of the woman being treated will also have some effect, as will the policy of the treatment centre concerning the number of inseminations to be undertaken in each cycle. It has to be admitted that the pregnancy rate achieved with DI is generally lower than that which would be expected with normal intercourse among fertile couples. The difficulty in timing the insemination appointment accurately to coincide with ovulation is probably a major factor in explaining this lower rate.

Care should be taken in interpreting success rate figures; they are statistical averages representing large numbers of couples and while they provide a rough estimate of the likelihood of achieving a pregnancy, they are only estimates. Much will depend on the circumstances surrounding the individual receiving treatment and the type of DI treatment provided.

The pregnancy rate per couple may well be affected by the fact that a considerable number of couples decide to give up DI, and some give up quite quickly before the procedure has had much chance to be successful. One study showed that 40 per cent of couples who gave up did so within the first five months of treatment. This suggests that these couples may have changed their minds about continuing with the DI treatment for some reason which may not have been directly related to a failure to get pregnant by DI.

Another problem is that of stress. Research has shown that psychological stress can cause the regularity of the menstrual cycle to become upset and thus cause disturbance to the timing and even the occurrence of ovulation. If cycles become irregular or ovulation does not occur, the accurate timing of insemination becomes very difficult or impossible. It is helpful, therefore, if couples can maintain a positive attitude towards DI. This is of course easier said than done, but if emotions get too intense they can work against a successful outcome of treatment. A more philosophical approach which can accept the result of DI treatment whatever the outcome is not only more healthy in itself but is also more likely to lead to the desired result. Even where a pregnancy is elusive, many couples find inner depths of strength in themselves and in each other that they had not previously known they possessed; this growth in their relationship can of itself be a worthwhile outcome of treatment.

The centre where DI treatment takes place should always be informed about the outcome of donor insemination. When a woman becomes pregnant it is very important that she tells the centre about this so that they are aware of the success of their treatment and can keep proper records.

If a pregnancy is achieved, how long does it usually take to conceive?

Some couples are under the mistaken impression that conception is likely after the first insemination, and are then very disappointed when this does not happen. Of course, conception does sometimes occur during the first cycle but the majority of couples who eventually become pregnant have to wait longer than this, often attending the centre for DI treatment over a period of several months. However, most women who do conceive do so quite quickly and research studies have shown that most conceptions occur within the first five or six cycles if insemination takes place during each cycle; that is, during the first five or six months of DI treatment. This leaves a minority of couples who, though they are eventually successful in achieving a pregnancy, take longer to conceive. If a pregnancy has not been achieved within the first six months then it certainly does not follow that all is lost. Many DI parents would argue it is often worthwhile persevering with treatment for a longer period.

As we have already described, psychological stress can sometimes delay conception. During our discussions with couples it was quite common to hear that conception occurred in a month when the couple were completely preoccupied with some other matter, perhaps the illness of a close relative, or a move to a new house. Once the couple were no longer preoccupied with conceiving and their minds were on something different, then a pregnancy was achieved. Perhaps there is something to be learned from this.

How long will treatment continue?

It is wise to decide with the doctor, right from the beginning, a reasonable time period during which treatment is to continue should a pregnancy not occur. The majority of conceptions occur quite early in treatment and most doctors would suggest that if conception does not occur within five or six months then a review of the treatment should take place to see why success is proving elusive. Perhaps investigations of the woman's fertility will need to be considered, or drugs may need to be prescribed for the better timing and control of ovulation. Some women become increasingly anxious to conceive and more disappointed and threatened by each month's failure, and uncertainty about how long a doctor will be prepared to continue treatment can cause additional stress. As explained previously, stress tends to work against the likelihood of a conception taking place. Some of the couples we talked with told us that after they had received DI treatment for several months without success they began to worry that the doctor might think further treatment was unlikely to be successful and refuse to continue. Most had kept this worry to themselves and not broached it with the doctor. The couples could have saved themselves a considerable amount of worry if they had brought their fear out into the open. It is always wise to voice any doubts and anxieties rather than to worry privately about them, as there is often no basis for the worry and a simple question may clear up the matter.

However, there does come a point when it is foolish and mistakenly stubborn to continue with DI treatment any longer, and it becomes necessary to accept that pregnancy is unlikely to occur. To continue DI treatment beyond a reasonable chance of success can cause great anguish and distress to no purpose, and there eventually comes a time when it is best for all concerned to acknowledge this. Every centre is required to have access to an independent counsellor who will be available to offer help and support if it is necessary to come to terms with a painful decision of this sort; a chance to talk through one's feelings and disappointments at this time can help couples to see the way ahead more clearly.

Should a woman receiving donor insemination treatment continue to work?

There is no medical reason why women should not continue to work outside the home during the time DI treatment is being received; indeed, it may well prove beneficial to undertake such work. To have wider interests can reduce the stress sometimes associated with childlessness and DI treatment and a job often provides an opportunity to interact with a wider range of friends and colleagues. One study has shown that women who were working outside the home during the period when they were undergoing DI treatment were slightly more likely to get pregnant than women who were not employed outside the home. On the debit side it can sometimes be awkward to arrange time-off to attend the treatment centre, especially if appointments are made for attendance more than once each month. However, the experience of the couples we have talked with indicates that employers and work colleagues are generally sympathetic and understanding about the need for regular absences from work.

Are there any health risks associated with donor insemination treatment?

DI treatment is generally a very safe procedure, however the onset of the AIDS epidemic has brought with it important implications for the provision of this treatment. Because the AIDS virus (HIV) can be carried in the semen of an infected person there are now rigidly enforced regulations concerning the selection of donors and strict procedures for the quarantine and checking of semen. Men in high risk groups for HIV are not allowed to become donors and men who are accepted are required to have blood tests to exclude HIV infection. It is known that HIV infection takes some weeks to show up in blood tests. To ensure that the semen is clear of this infection the donor's blood is tested just prior to the time when his semen is collected. The semen must then be freeze-stored for a period of six months and at the end of this period the donor must undergo a second blood test. If the second test is also negative then the semen in storage is known to be uncontaminated and can be used.

Some couples worry that an infection such as gonorrhoea could occur after insemination if the donor had a venereal infection which he did not disclose. There is virtually no chance of this happening as semen specimens are examined microscopically to assess fertility and so signs of infection would be detected at the same time. In the highly unlikely event of such an infection being transmitted, treatment with antibiotics is possible.

When conception occurs as a result of DI treatment, the usual risks associated with any normally achieved pregnancy are present but there is no evidence to suggest that particular problems are directly caused by DI treatment. As with all pregnancies, it is important that the mother-to-be attends for ante-natal care in the usual way.

6

The Semen Donor

Who are the semen donors?

Donors are not easy to find and one of the main difficulties in setting up a DI centre is the recruitment of suitable semen donors. It is no small thing to ask a man to donate semen which may be used to procreate new life—a child, or children, which will be his genetic offspring, but about whom he will remain completely ignorant and for whom he can fulfil no responsibility. The very act of producing the semen sample by masturbation into a sterile container to be delivered to the technician responsible for its freezing and storage, requires a level of commitment which often goes unrecognised. The donor may be required to abstain from sexual activity for a time before donation and he must also be willing to undergo regular blood tests (including HIV testing). Like blood donors, semen donors receive no payment for their services although expenses may be reimbursed.

It is probably true to say that the majority of donors are university, usually medical, students. Most centres are situated either in university teaching hospitals or in large cities where there is a medical school, so medical students provide a readily available source of recruitment. Medical students can also be contacted discreetly by a personal approach during their training. In order to recruit more donors, or to provide a greater spread of donors across the community, some centres have advertised for donors, either in the general press or in student journals and newspapers. This publicity sometimes results in unfavourable comment and it is therefore not surprising that most centres base their donor recruitment on personal contact.

Medical students are not the sole source of donors, however, and other groups of people with whom the medical staff at the centre have contact are also used. The fertile partners of infertile women who have been successfully treated are one such source. A general approach may also be made to the fathers of new-born babies who visit their wives or partners in the maternity unit of the hospital in which the DI centre is housed. Men who are about to undergo a vasectomy operation because their own family is complete may also be asked if they would be willing to donate semen before the vasectomy operation is undertaken. Other hospital workers or more general acquaintances of the staff providing the DI service are also sometimes recruited.

In accordance with the Human Fertilisation and Embryology Authority's (HFEA) code of practice, centres are required to provide donors with adequate information about what being a semen donor involves. Before accepting the semen the centre must obtain the donor's written consent for its storage and use. Should a donor subsequently have second thoughts about his role he has the right to withdraw this consent at any time. This need for the donor's informed consent recognises that donors need to consider the implications (for themselves and their families) of their involvement in donor insemination. The HFEA code of practice also requires centres to have access to an independent counsellor who is available to any donor who feels he would like to talk through the implications of his participation in this particular form of family building.

How is the suitability of a donor assessed?

The law (in the form of the Human Fertilisation and Embryology Act, 1990) requires that the person in charge of the DI centre is responsible for the recruitment and selection of donors and this has to be done in accordance with the code of practice of the HFEA. Donors must be between the ages of 18 and 55 years and must give written informed consent to the use of their semen in DI treatment. Donors who are in a high risk group for HIV infection or who are otherwise not in full health must not be recruited. Irrespective of their health status, all donors must be tested for HIV infection.

The most important qualification for a donor is, of course, that he should be fertile. Some centres have a requirement that a donor should already have fathered a healthy child by his own partner, but it is more usual these days for the donor's potential fertility to be determined by microscopic examination of his semen. Sperm must be present in the semen in adequate numbers, and must also be active and properly formed before a donor is considered suitable. In the case of some potential donors, semen which is highly fertile becomes damaged during the freezing process, and so the ability of the semen to survive freezing is also assessed.

The donor must also be healthy; in particular he must not suffer from a disease or disorder which could be inherited by his offspring. The donor's family history is also checked; that is, the health record of his close relatives is inquired into to make sure that there is no history of hereditary disease in his family. The donor must also have no history of an infectious disease which could be passed on to a woman during the process of DI treatment. A donor's blood group is also identified.

In addition to physical health, most centres require their donors to be of reasonable intelligence. It is questionable to what degree intelligence is inherited and can be passed on to the child, but it is essential that the donor should be sufficiently intelligent to understand the implications of his action in donating semen. It is also important that he understands the responsibility which falls on him to behave conscientiously and responsibly in donating semen. The honest reporting of any infection, and indeed the fact that the semen delivered by the donor is in reality his own semen, must be taken on trust by the treatment team. Centres are required to give careful consideration to the suitability of individual donors; this often requires a decision by the whole treatment team. Whenever practicable the potential donor's family doctor should be asked whether there is any known reason why the individual might not be suitable.

The same regulations apply to the recruitment of donors where the treatment centre arranges this for itself or where the centre buys in semen samples from another, usually larger, centre. Some centres are relatively small and the time, cost and effort involved in the recruitment of donors is out of all proportion to the size of the centre. These centres often have a contract to obtain semen samples from one of the major centres which has a larger supply than it needs to run its own DI service.

How often are donors used?

The number of live births which is allowed to result from donor insemination from one donor is normally limited to ten. While there is no obvious scientific reason why the numbers of births from each individual donor should be limited, the psychological reasons are more compelling. It is not difficult to appreciate that individuals who had been conceived by DI might be disturbed by the thought that they share the same genetic father with tens, or scores, of others. The donor's own natural children might also be similarly disturbed. Donors might also be psychologically affected by the knowledge that they may have sired so many unknown offspring. Some parents of children conceived by DI are bothered by a nagging concern that because the genetic father of their child is unknown the child could, by a tragic coincidence, marry a half-brother or half-sister. This is a most unlikely eventuality, but one which increases in accordance with the number of live births sired by an individual donor. This concern is one reason why the HFEA maintains a register of donors and of children born as a result of DI treatment; individuals who believe themselves to be conceived by DI can make enquiries to ascertain whether or not they are closely related to an intended spouse or partner.

In exceptional circumstances this limit of 10 children from one donor may be exceeded. Sometimes a couple who have already had one child following DI treatment might wish to have another baby using the same donor. If semen from this donor is still available, and if the birth will not exceed any upper limit which that donor has himself stipulated, the donor may be used again to help this couple.

How is a specific donor selected for each couple?

The treatment team will attempt to match the general physical characteristics of the donor with those of the infertile husband or partner. But at the present level of scientific knowledge about these matters it is not possible to predict or arrange in any detail the precise physical appearance of any child. The 'shuffling' of genes which occurs when a sperm and egg unite at fertilisation means that children are born possessing an almost infinite variety of characteristics and are all unique. Children within the same family may show an overall family resemblance but brothers and sisters are often, both in appearance and temperament, very different from each other. However, certain general physical characteristics can be matched with reasonable accuracy. These include certain racial characteristics, height, body-build and the colouring of hair and eyes. A donor of the same race will be chosen. Infertile couples from minority racial groups may have particular difficulty in obtaining DI as practitioners find it more difficult to recruit donors from these racial minorities. Height and body-build can be classified into general types; there is the tall, thin, rather narrow-boned type and the shorter, broader, bigger-boned type. This does not mean that any particular height or body-build can be predicted, but that general overall patterns of body-build tend to be passed on in families. Similarly people with dark-haired, brown-eyed characteristics can be differentiated from those with fair-hair and blue-eyes. At the first attendance at the DI centre, a member of the treatment team (usually the doctor responsible for the medical aspects of the treatment) will note the racial characteristics, height, body-build, and colouring of the male partner so that these can be used for the selection of suitable semen from among the samples in freeze storage. This is one reason why a meeting with both partners is helpful to the treatment team. Blood groups can also be matched, particularly with regard to rhesus factor compatibility.

At one time parents were anxious that the characteristics of the donor should be matched with those of the infertile partner as closely as possible in order to hide any suggestion that the resulting baby might not be genetically linked to both parents. Even though couples are now encouraged to be more open about DI, it would still be inappropriate for the appearance of their child to be so different from the rest of the family that the difference attracted special comment by others or produced a feeling of isolation in the child. Research into the adjustment of adopted children to their adoptive families has shown that the children fit in more happily and are better adjusted if their physical appearance is compatible with that of their new parents. Striking differences in appearance can lead to comments by friends and relatives which are hurtful to the child because they act as reminders of the child's different status. Whilst most adopted children do not want their adoption to be kept a dark secret, neither do they want it to be the subject of continual remark. They want it to be accepted and then forgotten about as something relatively unimportant. This process of their adoption being taken for granted is aided if the child's physical appearance is similar to that of their adoptive family. Similarly it is beneficial from the point of view both of the child conceived by DI, and the child's parents, that the child should have a physical appearance which blends in with other members of the family.

One word of warning: we have already noted that even in families where the children are the natural (that is, the biological) offspring of the parents, striking physical differences sometimes occur. The family formed by DI can be similarly affected. Whereas joking references to 'the milkman' can be laughed aside easily in normal circumstances, DI parents may find such jokes harder to take. They may also unreasonably suppose that the DI treatment centre made a mistake and that an inappropriate semen sample was used. The inherited characteristics of human beings, whatever the circumstances of the child's conception, are far more variable than is often supposed.

Will the same donor be used at every insemination?

There is no firm rule about this and the practice will vary from centre to centre. Some centres may be able to arrange for semen from the same donor to be available at each insemination, though they will not be able to guarantee this. In other centres it is unlikely the same donor will always be used. As we have just seen, donor matching is undertaken according to certain characteristics and it is the donor *characteristics* rather than an individual donor that are important in donor selection. Centres record this matching through the use of a code which not only identifies the donor characteristics but also specifies the individual donor used at each insemination without divulging his personal identity. This code is recorded in the treatment case notes so that the donor responsible for any pregnancy is known and statistics about the number of births for which he is responsible can be collected.

In order to be certain of the genetic identity of the baby resulting from DI treatment, it is a requirement of the code governing treatment practice that when more than one insemination is performed during any one menstrual cycle the same donor must be used at each insemination within that cycle. This applies even where the characteristics of two (or more) donors may be very similar. For the same reason semen from more than one donor must not be mixed in the same insemination. In addition to the need to know the genetic identity of a particular child and to know how many babies are being born from the semen of a particular donor, it is important to be certain who the donor is in case the unlikely event of inherited disease is discovered at a later date.

How much information will be given about the donor?

The treatment team and anyone else who may be involved (such as the HFEA inspection team) is required, by law, to preserve the anonymity of the donor. For this reason, access to relevant medical records, appointment lists etc. is severely restricted and all documents relating to the work of the centre must be secure. The maintenance of confidentiality and record security is one of the issues that receives particular emphasis during the annual inspection visit by the HFEA inspectors. Any lapse could cause the centre to lose its licence to continue providing DI treatment. It is evident that this matter is taken very seriously but it also means that there is no way that the couple who have had a baby by DI or who are currently undergoing DI treatment can discover the identity of the semen donor.

In this situation the couple has to accept on trust that enquiries have been made to ensure that the donor is healthy, fertile and of a broadly similar physical appearance to the husband or partner. However, some couples feel that they would like to know more about the donor; not who he is but the sort of person he is, his interests, hobbies, talents and aptitudes. At the time of giving consent to the use of their semen for DI treatment, donors are required to provide information about their health, age, race etc. and this opportunity is used to encourage them to write a short description of themselves, a kind of pen-picture which gives an overall impression of the kind of people they are and the kind of life they lead. Donors are reassured of their anonymity and do not have to provide this additional information if they do not wish to do so, but they are advised that this sort of information would be found helpful by interested parents or by any a child who might be conceived.

This descriptive (but not identifying) information should be made available to the couple by the treatment centre. Because the same donor is not invariably used at each insemination, the description of the donor is usually given to the couple when a pregnancy is established. This is a new practice and while some centres encourage the transfer of this type of information, not all do so. This is usually because the donors have decided not to provide this information or were not encouraged to do so. Sometimes appropriate administrative procedures are not yet effectively in place in the centre. It goes without saying that the more frequently couples ask for this information the more likely it is to become a routine part of the DI service in all rather than just some centres.

While the couple may themselves feel reassured by knowing something about the donor, this information is intended primarily for the benefit of the child. Parents are now encouraged to consider telling their child that he or she was conceived by DI and this is the sort of information about the donor which is thought to be of the most interest and help to the child. Research among adopted children has demonstrated that very few children show interest in knowing the actual *identity* of their biological parents, but frequently ask for information *about* them. It gives a child a more secure and confident sense of personal identity and worth to know that the donor as well as the parents with whom they live are all valued and valuable members of society.

Some couples may find it hard to acknowledge that the donor is a real flesh and blood person and may have a natural inclination to push him out of mind. However, this information about the donor is a very important resource for the child and it is our view that couples should find out all they can about him at the time of DI treatment. It is not always wise to leave this until it is felt there is a need to know; obtaining this sort of information many years later may prove difficult and frustrating.

Will the same donor be used for a second baby?

This will vary from centre to centre. Some centres may be able to arrange this if a supply of semen donated by a particular donor is still available. Donor sperm is now routinely deep frozen and can be stored for a maximum period of ten years so it is possible to use the same donor for the conception of a second or subsequent baby. However, many centres do not have their own long-term sperm storage facilities (or sperm bank) and as a result it may be difficult to guarantee that the same donor will be used in subsequent treatment, sometimes years later. Donors move on and the donor whose semen gave rise to the first pregnancy may not be available when a second pregnancy is desired. As noted earlier, if the only hindrance to use of the same donor is that his semen has already given rise to the permitted maximum of ten live births, then a special exception can be made where a couple particularly request that the same donor is used when attempting a subsequent pregnancy.

Many couples do not mind whether the same or different donors are used, but some believe that their children will have a closer feeling for each other and will get on better together if they are full 'blood' brothers and sisters. Whilst it is understandable that DI couples should want to approximate as closely as possible the situation present in the 'normal' family, it is not at all certain that having the same donor for both children would make them more likely to get on well with each other or even to look alike. It is likely that being brought up together in the same family environment is what determines the feelings of closeness and support that many brothers and sisters have for each other. Many fully related sisters and brothers also spend a good part of their lives quarreling and fighting with each other and it would be wrong to expect brothers and sisters conceived by DI to be any different.

Does the donor have any legal rights or duties concerning the child?

The donor has no legal rights over any child who may be born as a result of his donation. The anonymity of the donor is a two-way process. Not only is the donor's identity withheld from the recipient couple and any resulting child, the donor also has no access to the identity of the recipient couple. Nor is he permitted to know the identity of any children who are born as a result of his donation. In the same way that the donor does not have any legal rights over the child, neither does the child have any legal rights over the donor. There is however one exception. If a semen donor knowingly withholds relevant information about his medical history or his fitness to be a donor and this results in the birth of a child who has an inherited disability, then that donor can be named to allow the child to bring an action against him in a court of law.

7

The Couple and Donor Insemination Treatment

What should be considered when deciding whether or not to have donor insemination treatment?

Deciding to seek DI treatment is one of the most important decisions that any couple may have to face during their life together. The decision may result in the creation of a new human life, and the implications of that decision will therefore last not only for their own lifetime but also that of the child they will have created. It is important to take time to consider this decision very carefully and to avoid, as far as possible, reaching conclusions in a hurry and perhaps during a time of stress. In order to help couples make the best decision about DI, centres are required to provide access to counselling help. While centres *must* provide this facility there is no compulsion on any individual or couple to make use of it. In our view it is wise for all couples to take the time to talk about the implications of the decision to be made, whatever that decision may turn out to be, with someone who is skilled and knowledgeable and who is independent of those who will be directly responsible for providing the DI treatment. Doctors and nurses are always ready to answer questions but sometimes couples hesitate to ask because they worry that the medical staff are too busy and do not have time to be bothered with what to them might seem trivial concerns. Often it is not a matter of clear, straightforward questions which the couple need to have answered but a need to explore vaguely understood feelings that are hard to put into words. Above all, the counsellor has *time* to listen and discuss issues, no matter how long this may take.

Our advice is to seek out someone who is independent and can stand aside both from the couple's relationship and from the technical provision of DI treatment; a person who can be relied on to understand the emotional aspects of the decision to be made; a person who can keep professional confidences and who will offer guidance and comment in a creative and challenging way with no expectation of a particular outcome to the discussion. A trained counsellor is usually the best person to do this.

There are two main phases in the decision about whether or not to seek DI treatment. The first phase is that of accepting the fact of infertility. It is only when this phase has been satisfactorily negotiated that a couple can successfully move on to the second phase, that of deciding how to resolve their problem of childlessness. Infertility can cause a crisis in the lives of the individuals and couples who experience it; they may feel shattered by feelings of inadequacy and guilt, often accompanied by feelings of anger and resentment. Couples may also feel intense grief that the baby they had planned to have together—a baby that would be part of each of them—will now never be. While this turmoil of emotions and grief about infertility remains unresolved it is not possible to think clearly and constructively about the next step. A wise decision about DI cannot be made while there are still hidden feelings of blame and guilt and frustration which the couple find hard to acknowledge. These feelings about infertility must be resolved first. It is important that couples talk to each other, and listen to each other and try to be sensitive to each other's needs, so that they can recognise and accept each other's feelings about this intensely personal matter. One woman described the care she and her husband took about this:

> It was very upsetting to start with to realise we couldn't have children of our own, together. We sat down one night and we talked about it. We said, look, knowing this, it can either make or break our marriage. It could have broken it if we'd gradually drifted apart and not talked about every aspect. So we sat down and said we would discuss everything, and work at our marriage to make sure it didn't happen to us.

Once a couple have attempted to come to terms with infertility there is still the need for decisions about how to deal with the problem of childlessness. This also needs time and again benefits from good communication between the two partners. Often each partner may have been considering the possibility of DI without mentioning it to the other. Some women are hesitant to mention it to their partner for fear of hurting his feelings or provoking a hostile reaction. During our interviews one woman said to her husband: 'I didn't say anything about DI because I wanted you to say you wanted it. And then when you said you didn't mind, I said 'Oh, yes, I'd be quite keen.' Women quite often try to plant the idea of DI in their partner's mind without openly suggesting it. They say they are hesitant to broach the subject openly because they see the problem as being greater for their partner than for themselves. One woman said to us: 'To me I was getting everything. The baby was going to come with me; it would be more me than [husband], and I felt it was an awful lot to ask somebody. It seemed so unfair.'

All the couples we talked with stressed that the decision to employ DI must be a mutual one with both partners in full agreement. Each partner has to try to see the situation from the point of view of the other. This can be particularly difficult because the partners are not both starting from the same position. Whereas it is the male partner who is infertile, it is the female partner (who is both able and willing to bear a child) who receives the DI 'treatment'. One man described the decision he and his wife had made:

> We were both feeling each other out really, because I did not want to hurt her feelings and obviously she did not want to hurt mine. My wife said, was I at all upset about it being another man's, a donor. And also I had to ask her a straight question—did she mind it being another man's inside her.

As well as seeing DI from the point of view of one's partner, it is also important that each individual recognises what their *own* attitudes and feelings are; they must be true to their own judgement of what they honestly believe is for the best. It is unlikely that a decision to have DI will work out well if one of the partners is rushed into a decision by the other, or if one of the partners agrees to the procedure reluctantly or half-heartedly only to please the other. The time to express any doubts or misgivings is *before* DI treatment is begun—it is too late once a baby is on the way.

One final point: several couples told us they had come to a mutual understanding that if they ever had an argument or a row about any issue in their life together, mention of DI was absolutely taboo. DI was far too sensitive and potentially disruptive a subject ever to be used simply to score points in a quarrel. Once said, harsh or hurtful words about such a topic are unlikely to be forgotten; and once spoken they cannot be unvoiced. Even in the most heated disagreement there are some things best left unsaid if the quarrel is to be mended.

Is formal consent to donor insemination treatment necessary?

It is a legal requirement that a woman must give her written consent before DI treatment is begun. The written consent should explain the nature of the treatment and the steps which are to be taken. In order for her consent to be valid the woman must have been given comprehensive information about the treatment both orally and in writing. She should be given a copy of the consent form to keep.

There is no *legal* requirement to obtain a husband's or male partner's consent before treatment begins but the code of practice points out that the centre should make every effort to do so in the interests of establishing the legal parenthood of the child. While the centre will not be committing any legal offence by failing to obtain this consent, the licence to provide treatment may not be renewed if reasonable attempts have not been made to obtain it. A woman's husband or male partner will be the legal father of a child born as a result of treatment using donated sperm unless he can prove that he did not consent to the treatment. Centres therefore take all practicable steps to obtain his written consent.

This does not mean that DI treatment is only available to married women or women with an established male partner who is willing to take on the responsibilities of fatherhood should treatment be successful. Women who are not married or who have no male partner cannot be denied DI treatment solely on these grounds but the treatment team are required by law to ensure that account is taken of the welfare of the child who may be born as a result of the treatment, *including the need of that child for a father*. How this requirement is met to the satisfaction of those providing treatment depends on the particular circumstances surrounding each application for treatment.

Does donor insemination increase the risk of marriage break-up?

At the present time marriage break-up is a common occurrence in Britain; over one in three of all marriages end in divorce. However there is no evidence that couples who have had a child by DI are any more likely to divorce than other couples. Indeed it is sometimes claimed that the divorce rate among DI couples is lower than that among other couples. There is no hard evidence to back this claim as the treatment centres are not always aware of the subsequent experience of DI couples once their children are born. But some centres have attempted to keep in touch with couples following the birth of their children, and although not all couples have maintained contact, the general impression is obtained that divorce following DI is relatively rare. Our own contacts with DI couples over a period of 15 years supports this view. The factors which might account for this lower divorce rate are not clear and one can only speculate about the reasons which underlie it. It may be that couples who opt for DI are couples who are particularly committed to each other and who have the sort of relationship where they are determined to surmount problems and difficulties together rather than letting such problems destroy a relationship which they value. However we have no evidence, even of an anecdotal kind, which deals with the effect a discovery of infertility (as opposed to a decision to have DI treatment) might have on divorce rates—especially where the infertility is due to an incapacity in the male. There is an assumption that if a break-up of the relationship is to occur, it is more likely to take place before DI treatment is sought.

Several of the married couples we talked with told us that the husband had offered his wife a divorce when news of his infertility had first become known. These wives had dismissed such a suggestion. One said: 'He did ask me if I wanted a divorce—but I married him for *him*.' Another wife paradoxically explained: 'I said, "What do we want a divorce for? I want children, but I want *your* children, not anybody else's."' It should be noted that these couples were couples who had decided in favour of DI treatment. Had the wives acted on the husband's offer of divorce they would not have been reporting this conversion to us.

So it seems that couples who solve their childlessness by having DI, tend to be the sort of couples who value the quality of their relationship with each other and want to preserve and maintain it. It is possible that other couples who are less committed to each other take the option of divorce in preference to DI. If this is so, a lower rate of divorce among couples who have obtained DI treatment would be expected.

It would, however, be dishonest to suggest that couples who have DI never divorce. Some marriages do undoubtedly break up. In some cases perhaps these relationships would have foundered anyway and the experience of DI played little part in the break up; but in other cases friction associated with childlessness and DI has contributed to the conflict. Relationships are particularly likely to be damaged if the decision to seek DI treatment is not arrived at carefully and sensitively. If one of the partners has reservations and only agrees to DI treatment to please the other, these reservations can grow into grudges which gradually fester and spoil the relationship.

Will donor insemination treatment make any difference to our sex-life?

There is no reason to restrict sexual activity during DI treatment. Indeed, if couples are to maintain a positive and loving relationship with each other it is important that they should continue to have sexual intercourse in the normal way. The likelihood of successful DI treatment is increased if the person receiving the donor sperm is relaxed and contented. To avoid sexual intercourse while attending a centre for DI treatment is, if anything, likely to be counter-productive.

However, it may be helpful to know that when couples first learn they are unable to have children, some experience a temporary disruption of their sex-life. During infertility tests the husband may feel as though it is not only his fertility which is being examined and assessed, but also his sexual performance. There is often confusion between the ideas of fertility and virility; if the male partner discovers he has no *reproductive* potency, he may fear that his *sexual* potency is threatened also. In addition, when couples learn that they are unable to have children, sexual activity may serve only to remind them of this. They may feel that sexual activity has been rendered pointless by their inability to have children, and this feeling of pointlessness often helps to reduce normal sexual desire. In view of all this it is not surprising that many couples find that their sex-life suffers during the time when infertility is being diagnosed. Couples should not be unduly anxious about it, but should attempt to see these upsets as a fairly common reaction experienced by many couples. In the majority of cases these difficulties are relatively short-lived and once couples have got over the initial shock and have begun the process of readjusting themselves to the new circumstances, then sexual relationships tend to improve.

If the couple feels that they have more serious problems concerning their sexual relationship and are in need of help and advice it is possible to consult a specially trained and experienced psychosexual counsellor. The local family planning clinic or the family doctor will be able to refer a couple to such a service. Counsellors linked to the DI treatment centres will also be able to offer advice should sexually-related difficulties occur during treatment. Although couples may feel embarrassment at the thought of discussing such problems it is nevertheless sensible to seek professional help.

How do fathers react to their babies conceived by donor insemination?

One cannot of course predict how every husband or partner will react to a successful outcome of DI treatment but we can report that the men we interviewed had no regrets about their decision to have a child by this means. Most couples were aware that in some men the use of donor sperm could provoke a reaction of jealousy and rejection of the child and most couples discuss this together. It is interesting to note that all who raised this point in our interviews were confident that feelings of jealousy would not arise in their case. One woman said: 'I felt we had made this decision together, and we were doing it together—and so we both accepted the responsibility'.

However, when a pregnancy was confirmed some of this anxiety resurfaced and several men confessed to having a niggling worry that they might not accept and love the child when it was born. But this anxiety vanished as soon as the baby arrived; all the fathers we have spoken with say they experienced very profound and positive emotions at the birth of their children. There is no doubt in their minds that these children are theirs.

Many pregnant mothers make a point of taking care to ensure their partner felt included and involved in the experience of pregnancy. One woman said to her husband:

> We involved you in everything, didn't we? As soon as I felt the baby moving I let him feel it—everything. Just do it together. Whenever I had been to the hospital I'd tell him everything that had happened so that he never felt left out.

The majority of husbands or partners arrange to attend at least some of the antenatal clinic visits and are present at the birth of their children. Those who do this find that being present at the birth increases their feeling of participation in the process of creating their 'own' baby; which in turn helps them to establish a special bond with the new baby.

Several men expressed the view that DI had turned out to be a very positive solution to their childlessness. It allows their partner to bear her own baby which is more 'theirs' than would be possible with an adopted baby. One man said:

> It was second best obviously . . . The worst part was finding out that my sperm count was low. Once you've adjusted to that I don't really see how DI can be anything but hope.

It is possible for any new father to feel slightly jealous of a new baby even when that baby has been naturally conceived by him. This can happen if his partner takes over (or is left to cope with) all the responsibility for baby care and appears to have little time or energy left to spend with him. The whole family—mother, father and baby—benefit if the husband or male partner shares responsibility for some of the work of caring for the new baby. During our interviews we saw many fathers with their donor conceived children. We were impressed by how involved many of them were in the care and upbringing of their children and by the loving relationships which quite evidently existed between them.

But babies conceived by DI do of course grow up; several couples made the point that the period of the child's adolescence would be the most testing time. To love and accept a baby or young child is one thing, to continue that loving acceptance throughout childhood and particularly the period of adolescence often requires a level of stamina some parents find difficult to maintain. The problems and difficulties of being a father are not confined to DI fathers, but in DI they have an added element of difficulty because of the lack of a genetic link between father and child. The possibility of denying responsibility for a child's behaviour when family disruption occurs because the child is 'not really mine' has to be recognised and faced.

How do mothers react to their babies conceived by donor insemination?

It is not common for women who have become pregnant as a result of DI treatment to be worried about their own reaction to their expected child. Because they are bearing their 'own' baby they appear to have few worries about how they will react to it after it is born, though like all mothers-to-be they have occasional worries that the baby they are carrying will be healthy.

Of more significance is the anxiety women feel about the possibility of a negative reaction to the baby on the part of their partner. When we asked one woman if she had any initial worries about having a child by DI, she answered:

> I think the only thing was how he would accept the baby when it was born; you know, whether he'd reject it or whether he wouldn't. I was almost certain he wouldn't, but you had that problem there as to whether or not he would.

Another woman explained:

> I used to say to [husband] sometimes, 'It doesn't worry you, does it?'. It didn't worry me, but it worried me to think that he might be worrying about it.

Some women were bothered by the fact that they were going outside their marriage to have a baby; that another man would be involved. One woman who had resisted for several years her husband's suggestion that they should seek DI treatment because of his infertility, said:

> Well, to be honest I was absolutely repulsed by it. I'm married to my husband and it would be carrying someone else's baby. Really, in my mind, I was getting absolutely desperate for a baby, but I would in no way let that thought even be considered. It was all my fault that we didn't do DI earlier and I wish now that we had done it right away. But I'm one of these people that are very much governed by my heart, and if I had done it earlier I think it would have been wrong.

Other women were less concerned that the baby they were carrying was conceived by the use of another man's sperm, but minded more about it not being their husband's sperm. Although they wanted children, they wanted the children of this man they had chosen to marry, and some wives took a considerable length of time to accept that this desire would never be fulfilled. One woman said:

> I think secretly I still hoped that somehow, by some miracle, that I would have this baby by my husband—and so we didn't do anything about it. A couple of times we mentioned DI and then it would be forgotten.

If either partner has any uncertainty, it is important that the couple takes time to talk through these ambivalent feelings and attitudes and not rush into any hasty action. As we have said before, it is too late to have second thoughts once a pregnancy is established.

Does donor insemination in a second marriage present particular problems?

Many men entering into a second marriage do so without having had children in an earlier marriage. Sometimes the reason for the failure of the first marriage may have been due in some way to the man's inability to father a child. In such cases adequate discussion about the desire for children before the second marriage takes place is important. If this difficulty of infertility is properly talked out beforehand, the second marriage (leading sometimes to the arrival of a child conceived by DI) is more likely to be stable. After all, each partner now commences the marriage aware of what the situation is regarding the possibility of having children.

There are also couples who enter into a second marriage or relationship where the man already has children from a previous relationship, but he has had a vasectomy operation after the birth of the children making him unable to father more children. An unsuccessful vasectomy reversal operation may have been attempted or the couple may have had advice indicating that such an operation was not possible. This situation is different and in some ways more complex than the more usual circumstance of infertility. Here the currently 'infertile' male partner has already had children—and indeed still has children. If his second wife or partner is childless, her desire for children may be greater and more insistent than his. They may both want children to cement their relationship, and perhaps to equalise the standing of this relationship with that of the earlier relationship from which children resulted;, but it is always possible that the male partner will suggest, or agree to DI treatment more for the sake of his new partner than for his own sake.

His first partner will be aware of his vasectomy, and as successful reversal of this operation is known to be unlikely, she will also be aware of the likelihood that any children born in the subsequent relationship are the result of special treatment such as DI.

Differential feelings about 'step' and 'own' children may also cause problems. This is most obvious where the male partner's children of the first relationship are still living with him. The wife of a second marriage in this situation said to us:

> I react differently to [names of husband's children] than I do to [name of own child conceived by DI] since he has been born. Before he was born I convinced myself that I felt like a natural parent to my step-children, but since he was born I have been much more aware that I feel differently towards him than I do to the other children. On a practical basis I have less time for seeing to them. And emotionally as well I've less time for them, and its affected them. It is slightly easier for [husband] because he has known [DI conceived child] since the start whereas I didn't know [stepchildren] until they were seven, by which time they are fully formed individuals and you get to know them as people rather than as babies.

Anyone who has first hand knowledge of divorce knows that it is a traumatic and painful process. Divorce and remarriage produce family tensions and complicate personal relationships; when the complexity of DI relationships is added to the already complicated situation, the problems and hazards which can arise are multiplied. It is our belief that couples in this situation should think very carefully before undertaking DI treatment and should not look upon DI as an obvious or simple solution to their need for their 'own' children when naturally conceived children of an earlier marriage or relationship are present.

8

Being the Parent of a Child Conceived by Donor Insemination

What arrangements are made for antenatal care?

When a woman misses her period following DI treatment and suspects she might have conceived, she should notify the DI centre. The centre will usually arrange for an ultrasound scan to be performed to check whether or not a pregnancy has been established. If a pregnancy is confirmed she will then be referred by the centre for antenatal care at a maternity unit near her home. It is also usual for the woman's family doctor to be informed of the pregnancy.

The advice of the Fertility Committee of the Royal College of Obstetricians and Gynaecologists is that it is important for the woman to inform the antenatal team of the fact that the pregnancy has resulted from DI treatment so that the obstetrician and midwife know that this is a specially planned baby. Sometimes couples are hesitant about informing the obstetrician or midwife but if relevant facts are withheld from the team providing antenatal care this can lead to embarrassing and, more importantly, worrying situations. Sometimes information about the husband's blood group may be requested, or the dates of the last menstrual period and the possible time of conception may be queried if the size of the enlarging womb does not correspond with what would be expected from the dates, or if the baby's birth is overdue. The obstetric team cannot give the most expert care if relevant facts are withheld from them. The information about DI passed between departments will be handled in confidence; the code of practice requires this. Before the treatment team makes contact with anyone outside the treatment centre about a couple's DI treatment or its outcome, permission must be obtained from the person receiving treatment. The only exception to this is the central recording of the treatment and birth by the HFEA whose members, like the treatment team, are required to maintain the strictest confidentiality. Permission is usually obtained in writing at the beginning of treatment on a once for all basis.

Several couples we talked with pointed out the benefits of the obstetrician and the family doctor being aware that this was a very precious baby. One man said: 'I did feel that they were, if you like, a bit more on their toes. They realised how much was at stake and so in a sense, rather than an intrusion on privacy it was, paradoxically, reassuring.'

Are there any dangers to the baby when it is conceived by donor insemination?

There appear to be no additional physical hazards in being a DI baby; there is no evidence that DI treatment causes any increase in the proportion of handicapped babies who are born. Some couples are worried that the deep-freezing of semen may damage the donor's sperm and so increase the risk of an abnormal baby. Research studies have shown that there is no increase in the incidence of deformities in babies born following DI when freeze-stored semen has been used. Some of the sperm are damaged in the freezing process but these lose their fertilising power. Only the undamaged sperm, which survive the freezing and thawing process, will retain the potential of reaching and fertilising the egg. There are, however, risks inherent in every pregnancy, whether from natural conception or as a consequence of DI treatment. These include the risk of an ectopic pregnancy or of a miscarriage occurring. Miscarriage is always a most distressing occurrence, but a miscarriage after DI, when the pregnancy was such a longed for and striven for event, is particularly heart-breaking.

Although the risk of having a handicapped baby after DI is very slight and no greater than normal, it is nevertheless a possibility which couples should discuss. Some of the couples we talked with felt this was a particular worry. One woman said to us:

> I felt during the pregnancy that if the baby was handicapped it would be just too much. From my husband's point of view I felt DI was enough anyway—and for it to have been a handicapped baby would have been too much.

It seems to us that couples should not go ahead with DI treatment if they cannot accept the remote possibility of a handicapped baby. Babies are not possessions or commodities which can be ordered and then rejected as 'imperfect' if they are handicapped. Every baby is a unique human being of incalculable intrinsic worth, and with his or her own autonomous rights and individual value. If a couple wish to become parents then potential disappointments and even tragedies are a part of that role, along with the undoubted joys and fulfilment which parenthood brings.

Who is responsible if the baby has a disability at birth?

In every pregnancy there is a small risk that the baby will be born with an abnormality. Every expectant mother knows the occasional feelings of anxiety about whether the baby yet to be born will be 'all right'. The chances of any baby being born with an abnormality of some sort are very small and when this very rare but tragic event does occur it is very unlikely to be the fault of anyone associated with the care of the pregnancy; in almost all cases it is just one of those very tragic natural happenings.

Babies conceived with the help of DI are no different in this respect; there is the very small possibility that a DI baby, too, may be born with an abnormality. The treatment team who provided the DI treatment could in no way be held to be responsible for this, unless a doctor, nurse or technician had been negligent in some way. All reasonable care is taken to ensure that the donor selected has no history of transmissible disease, that correct insemination procedures are followed and that the freezing and storage of the semen is undertaken appropriately. The regular inspection of each licensed centre is undertaken in order to reduce to a minimum the possibility of human error. Despite this the parent has a right to make a claim against the centre if it is believed someone has been negligent when providing treatment; it would be for the courts to decide whether reasonable care had been exercised in the provision of treatment and/or the selection of the donor. A donor could also be held liable if he knowingly withheld information about his medical history or his fitness to be a donor.

How do parents feel about their baby?

In our contact with families we found that the majority of parents were deeply involved in the care of their children who had been conceived by DI and showed a strong commitment to family life. Because these children had been achieved often after considerable heartache and after much effort, they were particularly valued and loved and the couples tended to find parenting especially rewarding and satisfying. One mother said to us: 'I think they seem more precious to us—you take it for granted almost don't you, normally?'

In most of the homes we visited, toys were very much in evidence and the couple spent much of their time playing with and talking to their children. Many of the children seemed to be quite forward in their development and no doubt the stimulating environment which their parents provided for them at home was one of the reasons for this.

However, it would be a mistake to imply that parenthood is problem free. Our culture tends to encourage us to view motherhood through rose-tinted spectacles; advertisements portray pregnancy as serene and problem-free and motherhood as a state of blissful caring for a happily gurgling, sweet-smelling bundle of joy. This is not a true reflection of reality. A crying baby, and disturbed nights resulting in lack of sleep, can leave the parents feeling fractious and tearful too. Caring for a baby is hard work and demands a considerable degree of unselfish dedication, especially during the first few months. The rewards of parenthood are great, but the demands are also high.

Will the baby look like us?

As explained in Chapter 6 the treatment team will usually attempt to match the general physical characteristics of the donor with those of the male partner, but it is not possible to predict in any detail what the appearance of a child will be. However, many couples are anxious about what their baby will look like, and several women confessed to spending the last few days of pregnancy worrying if the child might have red hair, or an exceptionally long nose, or even by some awful mistake be of a different racial origin. Some couples are anxious about the baby's appearance because they feel they would prefer to keep DI hidden from everyone and they are fearful that a baby who looks very different from them will give rise to comment. Other couples whose family and close friends know that the child was conceived as a result of DI still prefer that the child should look like them because they understandably want the child clearly to 'belong' to the wider family group. When a new baby is born relatives, friends and neighbours all seem to feel obliged to pass comment on who the new baby resembles and this can cause couples to feel uneasy and embarrassed. One woman confessed:

> I find I swallow, and have to give myself a talking to, that they are not suggesting anything, that they are not prying or probing—it's just a natural comment.

One father who was describing his uneasy feelings when people were commenting on the likeness of his daughter pointed out that it made no difference whether the comments were negative or positive, saying: 'It's the same feeling when someone says she is like me as when they say she isn't.'

It would seem that anxiety over the likeness of the child is worse for couples who want to hide the fact that they have had DI treatment. Other parents are relatively unbothered about the problem; one young mother said: 'To my mind I'm not worried either way because she's healthy, and she's lovely, and she's ours—I don't mind at all.'

Similarity of appearance is not just a matter of physical structure. It can also involve mannerisms and expressions which are characteristic of the parent and which a child may observe and copy. Several couples pointed out that children had acquired many of their father's distinguishing mannerisms and so had become increasingly more like him as they grew older.

Do men see themselves as the true father of their children conceived by donor insemination?

Although all the fathers we talked with had accepted their children as their own, they still experienced some confusion about the paternity of their children. It was noticeable that in trying to explain their feelings about fatherhood, many of the men referred to the donor as the 'real father', although they were at the same time in no doubt that the child was 'their' child. One man struggled to describe his confused feelings about being the father of two sons conceived by DI:

> The fact that it was not mine—they are, I know they are mine—but it was in the back of my mind that it

> was never mine, never my child—I wasn't the one, the father—but I mean I know they are mine now, they always will be mine.

This confusion is to some extent inevitable. Although the husband or male partner is the legal father and is, in all practical terms, the father of the child, the person who provides for and loves and cares for the child, he is not the genetic father of the child. We may agree that the 'social' father is much more important in terms of practical fathering, yet it is a fact that the donor, a more shadowy and perhaps less important figure, is still the genetic father of the child.

The child has two fathers; a genetic father and a nurturing father. This paradox produces a contradictory state of affairs which couples find stressful, and which they feel needs to be resolved in some way. Most men do this by reassuring themselves that they are, in all practical ways, the child's father for they carry out all the responsibilities of fatherhood; the role the donor has played in fathering the child is, by comparison, unimportant. For example, the role of the donor is inevitably very brief; once he has delivered his semen for testing and storing his part in the action is complete. By contrast the fathering role of the husband is much more lengthy and enduring. Not only has he been close during the nine months of the pregnancy, he has also been very much part of the planning of the baby. As one woman who had successfully completed DI treatment put it: 'Apart from not putting the sperm there, [husband] has been there the whole time.' Some couples also emphasised the greater role of the mother in the pre-natal development of the child compared with that of the donor. One man said: 'As far as we were concerned the baby would be 99 per cent [wife's name] and one per cent lent from someone.' His wife expanded on this statement:

> That's always been your view, hasn't it? Which in a sense is true enough. After all the woman carries it for

> nine months, so its got to be more of the woman, hasn't it, if you look at it that way?

Couples also emphasised how important a part the husband or partner played in the upbringing of the child, in attempting to instill values and standards and providing a healthy and stimulating family environment. One infertile partner commented:

> I feel very strongly that we do impart more than the major part of the child, rather than it being hereditary factors. I believe the parents create the child rather than the child creating itself.

The fact that the donor is completely unknown as a person also diminishes his importance; there is no identifiable third-party who could one day make demands or who might cause embarrassment.

To acknowledge the fact that the child is the genetic procreation of another man is for most men a hurtful and difficult thing to admit. Some men find this admission so hurtful that they try not to admit it even to themselves. They tend to evade the issue through a claim that the child 'could well be' theirs. These men argue that the true identity of the genetic father is ambiguous; no one could possibly know for certain that it was not himself. He had continued to have sexual intercourse with his partner throughout the period of DI treatment and though previous semen specimens had shown no fertilising power, no one could be absolutely certain that this was so for every one of his ejaculations. One mother explained how her sister-in-law had remarked after the baby was born:

> You went up there for 18 months [before DI was successful] and didn't get anywhere, so who's to say that [husband] didn't come up trumps in the end? It's just as likely.

This is one of the ways couples appear to be helping themselves to feel more comfortable in what can only be described as an uncomfortable situation; a situation where the child's nurturing father is not his genetic father. It is natural for couples to do this. It is well known that most of us finding ourselves in an uncomfortable situation attempt to interpret that situation in a way that enables us to feel less uncomfortable.

But sometimes, when couples have not been able to work through their feelings about infertility, and to acknowledge their loss in not being able to have a baby together, the question of the child's paternity can lead to them blotting out from their minds any thought of the donor at all. There are several aspects to DI which lend themselves to this; for example, the clinical nature of the procedure. No man is apparently involved, only a doctor who, together with a nurse, has provided a medical treatment to deal with a medical problem. One woman receiving treatment emphasised this impersonality when talking to us: 'While I was pregnant it never entered my head—or I never really thought that it wasn't [husband's] child, because it's so impersonal.' Some couples assert that donor insemination is merely medical treatment. One man said:

> I can't even picture it as a donor to be honest with you. It's just a medical treatment the same as an operation is a medical treatment. It's the medical treatment for the medical problem, just the same as you take aspirins for a headache. I've got infertility, so you take DI to solve the problem that way.

If the woman is also having some difficulty conceiving with DI and needs additional treatment herself it is easy to see how this denial of the donor as a person can seem very plausible.

At first glance the idea of blotting out any thought about the donor and denying his existence—of convincing oneself, once pregnancy is confirmed, that infertility was merely a bad dream and that now all is 'normal'—seems very attractive. One mother attempted to explain her attitude about this: 'Once you are pregnant you're just like anyone else, so, what the hell, kid yourself—it's nice.'

However, denial has its costs. The unresolved conflicts remain, liable to re-surface again sometimes years later, perhaps when they are least expected and least wanted; and there always remains a degree of uncertainty and insecurity which can lead to tension and stress. Simone de Beauvoir wrote:

> Since we do not succeed in fleeing it, let us therefore try to look the truth in the face. It is in the knowledge of the genuine conditions of our life that we must draw our strength to live and our reason for action.

Denial of the true state of affairs and the pretence of normal conception is reminiscent of the practice followed by adoptive parents several decades ago. Since then it has been established that the emotional energy spent on denial and concealment is better expended in facing and resolving the problems which are inherent in adoption. Couples who have children by DI are now also encouraged to be more open about the way their children are conceived. This is not to say there will be no painful moments when facing up to reality; but avoiding doing so also leads to painful moments.

There is no doubt that there is also a straightforward forgetting about DI for most of the time, as DI treatment recedes into the past and ceases to be of current concern. This has the advantage of reducing stress and encouraging normal family relationships. Nevertheless, this forgetting is not complete and sometimes events occur or things are said which bring DI back to mind again. One couple who had told all their close family members claimed the family had accepted the situation without hesitation; the husband said: 'I think everyone basically forgets.' But his wife interjected:

> I don't think it's a thing that's constantly on people's minds—but it's not a thing that's totally forgotten either. People forget about it, it goes to the back of their minds, but it's never totally forgotten.

How should the birth of a baby conceived by donor insemination be registered?

Until 1990, when the Human Fertilisation and Embryology Act was passed, there was no legal way of registering the birth of a baby born after DI. In practice couples registered the baby by naming the male partner as the father of the child but this was, strictly speaking, against the law. The new Act rectifies this anomaly by stating that where a woman has conceived a child by DI the woman's husband or partner is regarded in all respects as the child's father (with one notable exception relating to inheritance of a title) unless it can be shown that he did not consent to his partner's treatment. Babies born as a result of DI are therefore registered in exactly the same way as babies who are naturally conceived.

Can parents who have had donor insemination treatment in the past get advice after the baby is born?

Sometimes couples may find they have a need to discuss problems, not only during the course of DI treatment but also later on after their baby is born. Couples are now encouraged to consider the need to tell the child that he or she was conceived by DI; they may well feel that they would like some advice concerning when and how this is best done. The counsellors who are available at all DI clinics to talk with couples having DI treatment would also be available to help couples later on with such questions as the children grow up. Like all babies, babies conceived by DI do not stay babies for ever but grow up into complex human beings. Parents may sometimes find themselves in a situation where they are unsure about what to do for the best. It often helps to discuss matters with a sympathetic third party, and couples should not be embarrassed to ask such people as their family doctor, a church minister, or perhaps a Relate (previously marriage guidance) counsellor for help if such circumstances arise.

9

Sharing Information About Donor Insemination Treatment

Should information about donor insemination be shared with others?

When DI was first introduced it was assumed by those providing the service and by most couples seeking treatment, that it was best to keep the whole experience a secret; only those directly involved needed to know anything about it. No one ever set out to explain in so many words why this secrecy was the best course of action. The decision to provide and use DI treatment in secret appears to have been based on the unspoken assumption that being open about the subject would be harmful in some way to those taking part and/or to the child born as a result of such treatment. In the main secrecy was just taken for granted and the basis for it not questioned. In the early days of DI provision in the UK—during and just after the Second World War—sexual behaviour was more strictly controlled than it is today and the DI procedure was extremely controversial. There was also considerable uncertainty about the legality of the practice, so it is perhaps understandable that in those early days both the treatment providers and their patients thought it best to say nothing about what they were doing.

But times have changed: now there is a greater amount of freedom in sexual matters; DI has attained medical respectability; legislation has provided a legal framework for its provision; and the registration of the birth of these special children provides both child and parent with the same rights and status as any other child or parent. There is therefore a much more relaxed approach to the sharing of information about donor insemination, and couples are now encouraged to be more open in their dealings with their child and with near relatives and close friends. The Human Fertilisation and Embryology Act also allows for the provision of a certain amount of information to children conceived by DI when they reach the age of 18 years. (See chapter 10)

But when discussing the more open sharing of information about DI we must be clear as to what information we are describing. The sharing or withholding of information about DI treatment has at least three separate components. First there is the *confidentiality* of the medical consultation between the treatment team and the couple. This confidentiality is a right which is considered to be essential to this, and any other, medical consultation; it is rigorously enforced in the code of practice which governs DI and there is no suggestion that there should be any relaxation of medical confidentiality in respect of DI. Second, there is the question of the *anonymity* of the semen donor; this also is rigorously protected in the 1990 legislation. There are two main reasons which underlie the policy of donor anonymity. One reason is of a practical nature; most DI treatment teams believe that men would be less willing to donate semen if there was any likelihood of their identity eventually being revealed to children who were born as a result of their donation. The other reason has more to do with the perceived need to protect the integrity of close family relationships in those families where the children are conceived by DI. It is thought that if contact occurred between the donor and the couple, or the donor and the child, conflicting emotional ties or tensions might arise. The most efficient way to avoid this contact is to ensure that the donor remains unknown. The third component of information about DI relates to how much the couple are willing to share knowledge of their recourse to DI treatment with their near family and close friends, and eventually with any child who might be born. It is this third component, which has traditionally been referred to as *secrecy*, which often creates the most anxiety and uncertainty for couples who have a child following successful DI treatment. Whereas in previous decades it was assumed that it was best for couples to keep knowledge of their treatment to themselves (and this was often encouraged by their medical advisers) the approach now recommended by the Royal College of Obstetricians and Gynaecologists is that couples should be encouraged to think seriously about sharing knowledge of their DI treatment with selected others and eventually to inform the child of his/her different origins. Couples are also advised to consider when to confide in other relatives as well as at what age to tell a child, and how this could best be done.

Couples are understandably concerned and anxious about what the response of others to knowledge of their DI treatment is likely to be. Our interviews with couples who have achieved a baby (or babies) in this way have given us the opportunity to see how they coped with this uncertainty. The first time we met the couples who talked to us about their experience of DI treatment was in the early 1980s, some years before the 1990 legislation was enacted; it came as no surprise to us that at that time just over one-half of the couples had decided to keep DI entirely to themselves, telling no-one about the DI treatment and with no intention of informing the child at any foreseeable time in the future. At that time there was much less general acceptance of (and knowledge about) the DI procedure.

Why do some couples feel they would prefer to keep donor insemination hidden?

In the main these couples want to put DI out of their minds, to pretend that it had never happened and to present themselves as a 'normal' family. As one mother put it: 'We just want to carry on as though nothing has happened.' At first this approach can seem to be very attractive, but it means that the tensions inevitably present in the situation have just been 'put on ice' and have not been resolved. Dealing with a situation by pretending it has not happened is hardly ever satisfactory because the situation does not go away and repercussions often have the unfortunate habit of resurfacing at the most unexpected and least wanted times.

This desire to appear as a 'normal' family points to the main reason why some couples decided to keep DI secret. They were afraid that others would be critical and think less of them if they knew their child had been conceived by DI; that is, they were afraid of being stigmatised. One man who expressed this fear of being discredited in the eyes of other people said: 'I don't like people to think that it's me—that I'm any less of a person because I can't have a child.' Couples were also sometimes afraid their children would be discriminated against if people knew of their different origins. On the whole individuals seemed to be reluctant to admit to a fear of stigma on their own account. Wives tended to express fears that their husband might be discriminated against, and husbands in turn expressed fears for their children. But after many conversations with these couples it has become clear to us that the main reason underlying secrecy is the fear that the husband or male partner would be stigmatised. One man was perceptive enough to remark: 'I think the basic [reason for] secrecy is the hidden psychological thing against my masculinity.' The majority of men who are discovered to be infertile find it very difficult to admit openly to their infertility.

Couples realise that DI produces a situation of imbalance with regard to family relationships. When a couple adopt a child, the child is not usually related to either partner who are to act as his or her parents, but in the case of the child conceived as a result of DI, 'blood' relationships are present on the mother's side of the family but not on the father's side. Therefore some couples thought that harmonious family relationships were more likely to be preserved if neither side knew anything about the child's different origins. Couples wanted to protect their parents from any distress, but they were also worried that their parents might be disapproving of their decision to have a child by DI. There was also a very understandable fear that if the child became aware that he or she was conceived by DI, the child's relationship with his/her father might be damaged, and the security and stability of the child itself might be put at risk.

It is important to notice that all the reasons for secrecy given above are only *fears*; parents were fearful that disapproval and damaging consequences *might* arise. They had no way of testing the reactions of other people without telling the secret, and once the cat was out of the bag there was no way of putting it back if reactions were hostile. In fact, those couples who have told their friends and relations have found them very accepting and supportive and the fears described above have proved unfounded—at least for them. The small number of children who were told have also coped remarkably well—but we will return to this later.

Clearly, there are parts of the lives of all of us which are ours to keep as private as we wish; it is right and proper that this should be so. However some information—or information which is withheld—has implications for other people which these people may feel they have a legitimate interest in, and a right to know about. This is especially so when those involved believe they have a trusting and honest relationship with each other.

Why do some couples prefer to tell their family and close friends about their use of donor insemination treatment?

We must remember that it was only just over one-half of the couples whom we first met in 1980 who had kept their recourse to DI treatment hidden from everyone. It is perhaps surprising that at that time, when medical advice was generally slanted towards keeping DI treatment secret, more than 40 per cent of the couples we talked to had told selected relatives or friends. Some couples did so because they felt their relatives had a right to know; it was natural to tell them. One man said:

> . . . because we are very close to them, and we've never had any secrets from them, we didn't think this should be a secret from them. They are part of the close family circle. . . So it just didn't dawn on us not to tell the family; there was no reason to keep them out of it.

Other couples felt they needed people to confide in and to share their problems with, and they valued the psychological support which these friends and relatives gave. For example one woman said: ' I'm very close to my mother. We talk about it and it makes it a lot easier.' Her husband added: 'You don't want to take all the burden on your own shoulders.' Another man said: 'I think to have made the decision to keep it totally to ourselves would have made it very difficult, particularly in the anxious times.'

Other couples did not want to become involved in deception and subterfuge; one couple told their family about six months after starting DI:

> It was getting so involved. I felt awkward having to sort of 'wriggle', if you know what I mean. When I came back they would say, 'How did you get on? Did she come up with anything?' and all this, and it got terribly involved.

There was also a feeling among some couples that it was not realistic in these days to imagine that other people would not guess that the couple were having DI treatment, even if they were not explicitly told. One couple who had told all their family about their DI treatment suspected that some close friends had also guessed that their child was conceived by DI; the wife said:

> . . . because they are friends that we've had for years, they have known of all the problems that we had, and I often wonder—I mean, people aren't thick. They must read the same magazines that I read, and whether they think to themselves, 'Mmm—I'm sure it is [DI]'. But nobody's ever said. It's a thing which I'm sure has crossed our friends' minds. It's crossed mine, because I've got a friend who is in exactly the same position as I am. She was six years trying for a baby, then all of a sudden out of the blue she is pregnant.

Basically these couples felt more comfortable and secure and at peace with themselves knowing that they had no skeletons in the cupboard. One husband, whilst acknowledging that to hide DI was possible, re-affirmed his belief that to be open about DI was the best way; he said: 'It [secrecy] must be harder actually. The way we are now, we're free at mind aren't we? We're free at mind.'

Does keeping donor insemination treatment hidden cause problems?

Most couples, whether or not they decide to be open about their DI treatment, find that keeping the treatment hidden has its drawbacks; some were left with a nagging feeling of disloyalty and felt generally uncomfortable about it. One man said:

> It just shows, in a way, you start a deceit or a pretence right at the start and you have got to maintain it. It is like any white lie or lies, it snowballs. That probably sounds more sinister than it is in some way. But it is true, you know in your heart that you haven't told everyone the truth, and if there is one thing to my way of thinking that is a drawback, it is that with DI.

Sometimes couples regretted the fact that they had concealed DI in the beginning; given the chance over again they would have been more open about it. It becomes progressively more difficult to tell relatives later on, because the couple then have to admit to withholding information and misleading the rest of the family in the past, as well as admitting to having DI treatment itself. One woman commented about her own and her husband's parents:

> I think if we had told them straight away perhaps they wouldn't have minded; but now I think they would think 'Why couldn't they have told us earlier?'

Some couples admitted that they felt uneasy at deceiving the grandparents about the conception of their grandchild; one father-to-be who was keen to share his joy of the good news of the forthcoming birth said:

> We felt a little bit uneasy breaking the news [of the pregnancy]. We had been trying for a baby for all this time. We went down to tell my mother and [wife's] mother, and we were watching their faces, and it passes through your mind, I wonder if they believe us? Do they know we are doing DI? I wonder if anyone knows?

Couples who were hiding DI from everyone found it necessary to conceal their visits to the treatment centre each month and they found there were difficulties about this. Often men accompany their partners to the centre and have to provide a reason for wanting time off work. One woman said: 'My husband had to take time off work. That's the most difficult thing about it; you do tend to get caught up in a lot of lies about where you are going.'

When couples are attending for a second baby the difficulty of keeping the visits to the centre secret is increased because arrangements have to be made for someone to look after the first baby. Many couples have to travel considerable distances to the nearest treatment centre and it is often difficult to take a baby or small child on these journeys. One mother explained:

> Although I could leave him [son by DI] with grandparents, it's difficult to explain where I'm going—you

> run out of reasons after a while. It's a big problem now. Sometimes you have a late appointment and by the time you get back it's past [the time] when all the shops have closed and parents say, 'Oh, where have you been?'

Many couples have been longing for a baby for several years and if DI treatment is not quickly successful they easily become very despondent and depressed by their failure to conceive. If they are not sharing the news that they are undergoing DI treatment this means that they have no one, apart from each other, with whom they can share their anxiety and frustration. This lack of sharing news means that the shoulders of others are not available to cry on. Just when a kind word and an understanding gesture would be most helpful they are cut off from the support and comfort of family and friends. Not only this, but these couples have to try to hide their feelings and appear as though nothing is wrong for fear of rousing suspicions in the same family members and friends. Some couples find this very stressful and wish that there was someone close with whom they could share their troubles. One woman who experienced this dilemma said: 'We've wanted to very much. There have been times when we've felt really desperate to talk to someone.'

Even in the joy of at last having the longed-for baby, keeping secret the nature of the baby's origin can still cause problems. When the baby is born, there are inevitably many comments about who the baby resembles and this can cause some couples to feel very uneasy and embarrassed. Some couples found that occasionally they were suddenly and unexpectedly confronted with a situation where they had to think quickly in order to cover their embarrassment or confusion. To others these may seem to be unimportant and insignificant occurrences, but for the couple the incident can take on added significance and become very important. One couple, who each had their own separate family doctor, had been referred for DI through the husband's doctor and the wife's doctor remained unaware. The wife described a visit to her own doctor:

> Just after the birth of the second baby, he did the postnatal check up and he said, 'What sort of contraceptive are you going to use?' And he could see I was looking a bit stunned, because I hadn't thought about it you see, that he was going to ask me this question. And I thought, 'Really, this is ridiculous. Am I getting just too stupid?' But still, at the same time, I couldn't tell him.

Other women have mentioned that they are sometimes put on the spot by women friends wanting to discuss and compare their experiences and decisions about contraception.

It is clear that for many of these couples, attempts to hide their involvement in DI treatment had caused a variety of problems. It would seem that attempting to sustain a family secret of this sort has many practical and psychological disadvantages.

How do family and friends react when they are told about donor insemination?

When a couple's parents learn that the couple are unable to have children owing to the infertility of either partner, they are usually very concerned and feel extremely sorry for both partners. Sometimes this unexpected news comes as a great shock to the parents; the mother of the infertile male partner is often most hurt by this unwelcome news. Care and sensitivity need to be exercised when sharing this information especially when there has been not the slightest indication that infertility might be present. But once the initial shock has passed the parent's usual reaction is to attempt to give comfort and do what they can to help soften the blow for their son and his partner. When they come to realise that DI treatment is probably the only means by which the couple are going to be able to have a baby of their own, almost all grandparents begin to see DI treatment as a solution to the problem rather than DI itself being a problem. Couples have told us that once their parents had had time to think about DI more clearly they were able to see its advantages and to overcome what initial prejudices they might have had against it. One daughter reported a conversation she had with her mother about this:

> I said to my mother, 'We're thinking about DI; you do know what that means?' So she said 'I think so. You won't have that done will you?' and then she thought about it for a second and said,'Well, of course, really it's better than adoption.' And then she rallied round. It was just the initial shock I think that we were doing something that they [the grandparents] hadn't thought about.

Another daughter, who was pleased she had told her parents and would do it the same way over again, said:

> My mother and father—they certainly had never heard of it. I think they found it a bit difficult at first. They're in their seventies—there's a definite generation gap. I think now they think it's wonderful that it can be done. My mother isn't one of these people who thinks having children is the be-all and end-all, but she knew we wanted children and they are very pleased.

Some couples have reported that the idea of DI had been suggested to them by their parents or another member of the family who had happened to read an article about it or had seen the subject discussed in a TV programme.

Sometimes couples had broached the subject with their parents rather warily as they suspected their parents might disapprove. One married man whose parents had known for some time that he was infertile said:

> I told my parents that we were considering this—with some trepidation. My mother is a very staunch

churchgoing lady and I thought, 'How is she going to view this?' I said 'We've decided to start a family' and she looked at me a bit old-fashioned and said, 'Oh, yes', and looked very interested to see how I was going to follow that one! And so I said there was a procedure called donor insemination, and we told them, and I waited for the grunts of disapproval, and her disappearing from the room in a huff—but I was rather surprised. I don't think they had any misgivings at all—in fact they expressed quite an interest in it, didn't they? My father was always very willing to drive [wife] down for her appointment.

On the whole couples are less hesitant about telling brothers and sisters. Perhaps this is due to the absence of an obvious 'generation gap' and the belief that people of about their own age will be more open to accepting the idea of DI. Often couples do not tell their parents because there is no way of testing their reaction, and if it turns out to be a negative reaction they are likely to regret ever having mentioned it in the first place. But we have not met with a single couple who had had a hostile reaction from their family or friends; one couple who had told several friends and relatives wrote: '. . . we received only positive encouragement.'

When is the best time to talk to others about donor insemination treatment?

The longer sharing the news is left, the harder it becomes to tell others. If close family and intimate friends are not taken into the couple's confidence right at the beginning of the news of infertility, then the openness on which these relationships and friendships are built can become strained and false. While the decision not to tell others at the outset may be due entirely to the couple's uncertainty about how the news of DI will be received, their reluctance might be interpreted as a lack of trust.

Because DI treatment might not be successful (and so perhaps there might never be a need to tell) it is understandable for couples to want to delay informing others until a pregnancy has been confirmed. While this is better than leaving the sharing of this news until even later, it does mean that couples cut themselves off from the support which family and friends can give during investigations and treatment. For this reason alone it is helpful to tell others as soon as infertility is diagnosed. The strength of the emotional and practical support they receive from others often comes as a pleasant surprise to couples. This is especially welcome if support is needed at a time of stress and not just when there is a successful outcome to treatment.

How do grandparents react to grandchildren conceived by donor insemination?

The couples we have talked with whose parents were aware of DI reported that their parents have accepted their DI grandchildren wholeheartedly, and show love and pride and delight in the usual way. One mother said: 'The grandparents treat the child just the same as any other grandchild—they thoroughly spoil him!' Once the child is born the fact of DI tends to fade into the background and is forgotten about for most of the time. Another mother said: 'I don't think they [the grandparents] even think about it now. I don't think it occurs to them—it doesn't even to us.'

Some couples point out that once the child is born he or she becomes a child in his/her own right and genetic origins became relatively unimportant. One mother explained:

> There doesn't seem to be any noticeable difference or distinction at all [in the grandparents treatment of the DI grandchild]. I think once the child has arrived you just take the child as it is.

This couple also had a foster child whom they were hoping to adopt and their own parents had also accepted this boy as a grandchild.

> In some ways it made me feel slightly easier about it, that she [the child conceived by DI] would be accepted by everybody, because he [the foster-child] has been so totally accepted—and I mean he was nothing to do with any of us at all!

Is the father's family likely to react differently from the mother's family?

Having a baby by DI means that 'blood' relationships with the child are present on the mother's side of the family but not on her partner's side. This causes a situation of imbalance in relationships and some couples are worried that the man's side of the family may feel at a disadvantage and be less attached to the child conceived in this way. Because of this couples are sometimes more uncertain about the reaction of parents and other family members on the man's side when compared with those of the wife or female partner. This affects the willingness to be open about DI treatment to either set of relatives. Some couples also worry that the mother's side of the family might feel unduly possessive of the baby because the baby is the genetic offspring of their daughter and not that of her partner. In our experience, almost without exception, the father's side of the family has reacted in a similar way to that of the mother's relatives. One couple described how both sets of grandparents adored the child and how it had made no difference to the way they had treated the baby.

> [Husband's] mother—if you're going to be personal, she knows it's not his child—she idolises the boy, doesn't she? We'll go out there for lunch tomorrow and I'll lose the baby. It's lovely really.

In only two cases have we come across couples who have felt that the paternal grandmother had tended to hold herself slightly aloof and had seemed rather uninterested in her grandchild. But in both these cases other tensions in the family were reported by the couple, who also stated that they did not feel the paternal grandmother's attitude was entirely due to the experience of DI. This illustrates a very important point; all families experience stresses and strains at times; infertility and DI should not be seen as the lone cause of such tensions, but in the context of the usual experience of occasional family upsets.

Concluding remarks: sharing information about donor insemination treatment.

It must be obvious from the information we have presented in this chapter that we believe the inclusion of close family members and friends in the decision to have DI treatment is an appropriate and wise course of action to take. We also believe this course of action to be beneficial to all concerned. Trying to keep DI treatment hidden from others can have serious disadvantages; it implies there may be something shameful about DI, something which cannot be talked about and should be hidden for fear of arousing disapproval. While such fears may have had some justification in years past, the changed social climate means this is now less likely to be the case. Hiding DI from close relatives destroys the trust on which all good family relationships are built, especially where secrecy would lead to the deliberate deception of one's own child. It may not seem important for a baby to be told the truth about its different genetic origins, but that baby will grow up to become an adult man or woman. An adult is likely to feel cheated if he or she has been deceived about his/her origins. Add this to the psychological cost to the parents of attempting to maintain a life-long secret and there is a high risk, sooner or later, of experiencing emotional disruption and personal regret.

Many of the couples we have talked with who elected to hide their DI treatment did so because they feared what the reaction of others might be. The experience of couples who had shared the knowledge of DI with close family and friends would suggest that these fears are exaggerated or even groundless. Their confidants had been understanding about the situation and had offered wholehearted support and encouragement. Families had greeted the arrival of their grandchildren, or nieces or nephews, with the usual pride and delight and the children had been lovingly accepted into the family circle.

Nevertheless, the couples we have spoken with generally recognise the need to approach this topic carefully. Older people must be given time to let the information settle. The news of infertility and the possibility of DI treatment is likely to come as a shock and their immediate unconsidered reaction may be negative. First reactions of this kind are usually modified when the older people have had time to consider. After all, if young people (who supposedly have a less conservative view of new or controversial procedures) need time to accommodate to the idea of DI, then an older generation is even more likely to need time to adjust to these new medical treatments which go far beyond anything they could have experienced. If support is not offered by family members—though our experience shows this to be unlikely—the couple have the satisfaction of knowing they have been honest and have behaved with integrity. These are the very values most of us would like to pass on to our children, whatever their genetic background.

10

Children Conceived by Donor Insemination

How do the provisions of the 1990 Human Fertilisation and Embryology Act affect a child conceived by donor insemination?

The ultimate and sole purpose of DI treatment is the eventual birth of a healthy baby. Yet in the complexity of decisions to be made about treatment, and in the attempts to solve the problems of the infertile couple by successfully achieving a pregnancy, it is all too easy to forget the needs of the child who will be the result of all this endeavour. This is not so surprising as it might sound as the infertile couple are the doctor's immediate patients and at the time of DI treatment the child does not yet exist. The legislation which underpins the provision of donor insemination stresses the importance of considering, right from the beginning, the needs of any child who might be born. The Human Fertilisation and Embryology Act 1990 specifically requires that '. . . A woman shall not be provided with treatment services unless account has been taken of the welfare of any child who may be born as a result of the treatment (including the need of that child for a father), and of any other child who may be affected by the birth.' The code of practice which regulates the provision of DI gives guidance to the treatment team by setting out a list of factors which affect the welfare of the child and which should be considered before any treatment is started. These factors include such things as the ages and medical histories of the couple seeking treatment, the commitment of the couple to having and bringing up a child and any risk of harm to the child.

The Act also provides for a certain limited amount of information to be made available to individuals conceived by DI who may make enquiries when they become adult. At the age of 18 a 'child' can make application to the Human Fertilisation & Embryology Authority to find out about his or her origin by donor insemination. The applicant must be given a suitable opportunity to receive proper counselling about the implications of this request, and only non-identifying information about the donor may be made available. For example, if marriage is contemplated the applicant may wish to check that there is no risk of being a half-brother or half-sister to the intended spouse. (This information can be given from the age of 16 years if a minor is intending to marry.) Such a situation might arise if both have the same genetic father. While only non-identifying information about the donor would be provided, the applicant would be informed if there was a biological relationship with the intended spouse which would prohibit marriage.

Non-identifying information about the donor is also available to the couple at the time of treatment. In addition to physical details such as race, colouring, and height, donors are encouraged (but cannot be required) to provide some anonymous biographical details which can be passed on to the couple. This information is intended to be of assistance to parents when explaining to children about their donor conception.

Balancing the needs of the child with the needs of the couple can raise some conflicts of interest. What is seen as being most desirable from the couple's point of view is not always the most desirable when seen from the child's viewpoint. Maintaining the anonymity of the donor, as the 1990 Act does, poses such a conflict of interests. Some couples might feel very threatened by a proposition that their child should one day be able to learn the identity of the semen donor. However, many professionals working with children believe that the present institutionalised restriction on their knowledge is not in the best interests of the children concerned and will prove very frustrating to young adults who learn that they were conceived by DI. It is understandable that young people might well be made angry and frustrated by the knowledge that 'bureaucracy' holds identifying information about the donor, information about their own biological identity, but this is purposefully being withheld from them.

However carefully the best interests of the child are protected it seems to us that it is wise to admit that DI treatment may sometimes require a child so conceived to have to cope with difficulties over and above those of a naturally conceived child. Whilst DI might be seen as a solution to the couple's problem of childlessness, it must be acknowledged that DI holds the potential to be the source of problems for any resulting child. Couples considering DI as a means of solving their childlessness will need to balance their desire for a child created in this way against the weight of possible problems which might lie in wait for the potential child. Much will depend on an honest appraisal of their resources and ability to help their child cope with any such problems. This is an area which a couple should discuss very carefully with each other and perhaps with other close family members before deciding on DI treatment. The help of a skilled counsellor can also be invaluable.

What is the legal status of a child born as a result of donor insemination?

Before 1990 the legal status of a child conceived by DI was confused and uncertain. The Human Fertilisation and Embryology Act remedied this situation and provided a legal framework for the birth registration of such children. The legal status of a child born following DI is now similar to that of naturally conceived children. There is just one exception; a child conceived by DI cannot succeed to an hereditary title. The husband or partner of the woman undergoing DI treatment is regarded in all respects as the child's father unless he can prove he did not consent to his partner's treatment.

Do parents normally tell their child that he or she was conceived by donor insemination?

Before DI treatment became generally accepted by the medical profession, and when there was considerable uncertainty about the legal status of a child conceived by DI, couples were almost always advised not to tell the child of his/her different origins. However, the conditions under which DI is now provided have changed; the procedure is relatively common, it is an accepted medical procedure and a legal framework has been put in place which protects the status of the child. In the light of these changes couples are now advised that it is wise for them to consider telling the child. A policy report on infertility counselling concluded: 'Prospective parents need to consider the child's need for information about his/her genetic origins .... There is a considerable body of research evidence which demonstrates the importance of openness and honesty in family relationships.' In a similar vein, the Fertility Committee of the Royal College of Obstetricians & Gynaecologists advises: 'The couple need to consider seriously telling the child of the nature of donor insemination, the age at which this might be done and how it might be presented.' And the code of practice governing DI treatment advises those providing DI treatment: 'Where people seek treatment using donated gametes (i.e. donated sperm or eggs) centres should take into account a child's potential need to know about his or her origins and whether or not the prospective parents are prepared for the questions which may arise while the child is growing up.'

But even with official advice on which to rely, deciding what and when to tell a child can be very daunting. The couples whom we have known since 1980 had their children at a time when it was generally accepted that children would not be told. Despite this several couples were uncertain what to do for the best and found the decision of whether or not to inform their child a worrying and perplexing problem. The comment of one mother demonstrates this uncertainty:

> I'm not sure what I will do. I don't know, I'd discuss it with [husband] first anyway. That is a big problem. I wouldn't want to tell him [child] actually—that's the truth of it.

After a long pause she added:

> The problem will be when he is older, he may find out, we might have to tell him. We are pretty open with him. Well, if he's brought up the right way, and we hope he is, it won't make a bit of difference to him.

Couples who followed the advice of the time not to tell their children said they were afraid the children would be distressed by the knowledge that their father was not their father in all respects. They were also afraid that the children would be disturbed by a feeling of uncertainty about their own self-identity; this would be due to the fact that the donor who gave rise to their conception remained anonymous. They feared their child might be stigmatised at school and taunted by other children. There was also the recognition that telling the child about his/her DI origins might be hurtful to the child's father as well as to the child; the child might think less of the father or even reject him altogether. These reasons against telling the child were based on fears of what *might* happen. Often the fears of the unknown or what *might* happen are far greater than the actual stress in coping with a real situation. Indeed what we anticipate as stressful sometimes turns out in reality not to be stressful at all. The reactions of some young people who were told of their DI origins (described later in this chapter) tend to support this view.

Paradoxically, many couples, after they had detailed what potential harm knowledge of DI origins could do to a child, also acknowledged that they thought their child would be able to cope with such news. One father, when describing the resilience of his son conceived by DI, said:

> In our circumstances I don't think it would [cause] harm somehow. It would be a shock, but he gets so much love and attention from both of us that I don't really think it would make a lot of difference.

Despite contrary advice, some of these couples who now have children in their teens decided from the very start they would tell their children of their DI origins. The couples who had told their whole family and their close friends thought it would be preferable for them, the child's parents, to tell their child rather than for this information to be learned accidentally from others. One man saw this clearly:

> I think we will have to tell her because of the fact that our family know, because otherwise the chances are that it will come out, not intentionally, but it could come out. She should hear from us as opposed to hearing from someone else.

Some couples felt that the child was entitled to know and it would not be fair to keep a child in ignorance of his or her origins.

> The health visitor said there is no real need to tell him, but I think I will have to wait till he is older to decide. I'd like him to know really, I think we ought to be honest with him. I don't think its fair on him not to tell him, because if he has grown up with [husband] as dad, then he's always going to think of him as dad.

Some couples realised that as the child grew older circumstances might change and they might have to consider telling the child later on if the need arose. One father said: 'I think if for some reason he ever did think there was something up, if it was on his mind, I'd talk to him about it.' Our interviews with a smaller number of older couples whose DI children had all now grown up and left home, confirmed the suspicions of some younger couples that circumstances might well change as the children grew older. These older couples had not initially planned to tell their children, but some of them had found that as the children grew up, unexpected and unpredictable factors cropped up which made them change their minds. The older couples who had told their children had done so because they felt it would be beneficial for them to know. The children had had problems of various kinds which the parents believed would be alleviated if they were told about their DI origins.

Sometimes children ask questions which unexpectedly turn out to be awkward to answer. For example, children who are studying biology at secondary school have lessons about genetics and the inheritance of characteristics. This study is at an introductory level and might not always be well understood by the child; but sometimes such study prompts the child to discuss or question at home the characteristics (particularly eye colour) which they have inherited from their parents. Even if the child's grounds for questioning their parentage in this way are entirely innocent, the fact that the matter has been raised can cause the parents to feel insecure. This has happened to parents who have had children following DI treatment. An older man described his reaction when one of his sons had asserted that the colour of his eyes could not have been inherited from his mother and father.

> While they were young I was only too proud and pleased to have felt that the children were mine, and nobody ever enquired or said, 'They're not your children', or anything like that. So all the time they were juniors I felt confident that nobody would query it. It was not until the later date that my son came up with this at the age of 14, that I couldn't be his father, that it all started ticking over. And I thought, well, eventually I will have to tell them . . . Because, I mean, [wife] never felt that side of it because she regarded the children as hers all the time. But it was different

> for me. I knew inwardly they were not mine. But the children didn't know that—I did. So I felt should the occasion ever have to come out, then it must come out in the open.

Although these particular sons were not told of their origins at the time of this 'eye colour' incident, they were told a year or two later and it is clear that this episode had considerable influence on their parents' decision to tell them.

Every individual couple must of course make their own decision about whether or not to tell their child of his/her different origins, but there are good reasons why couples are now advised to be more open. Children tend to be very aware of undercurrents about things which are *not* said and subjects which are *not* discussed, and they are often very quick to pick up unspoken messages. They may not feel able to voice their suspicions and uncertainties openly, perhaps because they are aware that this is something that is not talked about, but their uncertainty and insecurity may well remain a problem for them. Not to tell the child about his or her genetic origins means that the child is being deceived in certain important respects and the parents are never being fully open and honest with their child. A couple may feel that they are withholding the information in the best interests of the child and to spare him or her from being hurt. However, the research and observations of those who work with children has shown that children are less upset by strange and apparently unpalatable facts than they are by any form of deception. Children can cope with unpleasant or difficult situations surprisingly well, but they need a secure and consistent base and they must be able to trust people, especially their parents. Not to be honest with a growing child is, to some extent, to deny that child the sort of respect to which each of us believes we have a right.

Thirty or forty years ago couples who adopted children were also reluctant to tell these children that they were adopted. But as adoption has become a socially accepted procedure, so it has become usual for adopted children to be told of their adoption. Although adoption is different from DI there are also some similarities between the two procedures; they both present a situation where there is a dislocation between genetic and nurturing parenthood. But in the case of adoption this is usually present for both parents, whereas it is present only on the father's side where a child is born following DI treatment. Experience with adoption has shown very clearly that adopted children fare better when they are told the truth about their biological origin, provided they are told in a planned way by people who love them and care about them and who respect how they feel. It is reasonable to assume the same is also true for children conceived by the use of donated semen.

Some couples who are reluctant to tell their child of his/her DI origins recognise they are also influenced in their decision by a desire to protect the husband or male partner. In telling the child, the man's infertility would be acknowledged and once the child was told about DI it would be possible others would also learn about his infertility. This can be a daunting prospect for some men. It is important to understand that being open with the child but hiding DI from everyone else is not a realistic option. It is possible that a child would tell other people; but it would be damaging to the child to expect him/her not to speak of it to others. To give a child some information which he/she is then told not to divulge to anyone is to suggest the information is in some way discreditable. As this information is about the child's own origins and self-identity it is easy to see how this might lead the child to feel personally discredited in some way.

One last point about this matter. To tell or not to tell others is not an 'all or nothing' decision. The alternative to total secrecy is not a public—and publicised—statement about one's infertility. Being open about a particular condition does not mean that it *must* be discussed with everyone. For example, many men and women have had an experience of divorce these days, and although this is not usually kept secret in a particular case, it is a subject that is not spontaneously raised. However, should a situation arise where reference to a past experience of divorce seems relevant or helpful, there is no fear of mentioning it. A similar situation has been reached in relation to the experience of adoption. It is to be hoped that it is only a matter of time before this will also be true of DI treatment.

Could a child find out accidentally that he or she was conceived by donor insemination?

In the early days of DI provision it might have been possible to keep knowledge of a child's DI origins from the child with little fear that this knowledge would accidentally emerge. Very few people had heard of DI. But in recent years DI (along with other forms of assisted conception) has become more commonplace. What is more, this topic is now widely discussed in the popular press and on radio and TV. This means that children who are growing up today are bound to be much more aware that some children are born following the use of such techniques. They are very likely to be curious to know if this applies to themselves. In the same way that many growing children ask their parents 'Am I adopted?', it is not difficult to imagine growing children asking their parents, 'Am I a test-tube baby?' Many parents tend to dismiss as unlikely the possibility of their children finding out from people who know even when several friends and relatives have been told: 'I don't think they would ever tell; it never comes up in conversation.' Virtually everybody had told *someone* about their need for treatment, even if their partner did not know of this sharing of information. Though couples may believe that only specific people whom they have told are aware of their child's donor origins, it is of course impossible to say how many people actually know. There is for most people an almost irresistible urge to share information with at least one other confidant. The network of people who have been told at some time is likely to be much wider than parents think. In addition, other children in the family, perhaps cousins, might well overhear parts of adult conversations and then discuss what they have heard with the children concerned. It is known that the sharing of family secrets is most often accomplished through the interaction of young cousins, often of the same sex and age.

We have found that although parents might never refer explicitly to DI, they do make indirect allusions to the topic. Comments to a child such as, 'You've always been expensive, even before you were born', may seem to be quite innocent at the time but comments such as this are often pondered upon and speculated about by children. One couple reported that if comments about the likeness of the child to her father were made by other family members or friends: 'We have a little private smile'. Such smiles are unlikely to go completely unobserved and it is very likely that children will be aware that something lies behind such hidden messages; as one mother commented: '. . . And children are very astute—they can hear things round corners!'

Couples also realise that if a child is not told by choice at a young age, it is possible that he/she could be told in anger, perhaps in the heat of a family quarrel during rebellious teenage years. One man put this very clearly:

> That still does concern me, actually. I suppose it's the point of concern that adoptive parents have, that when you get to adolescence and the balloon goes up as it were, it's easy to shelve off responsibility by perhaps even in anger actually saying, 'Well he isn't mine anyway. This is nothing to do with me.' And it does worry me that one hopes one is going to have the equanimity and stability to weather any storms of that kind.

There can be no certainty that because older children do not confront their parents with their vague suspicions that they have been conceived 'differently', they do not suspect this might be so. Adoption research has shown that children who find out accidentally that they are adopted frequently do not feel able to tell their parents what they have been told. It may well be that some of the grown-up children conceived by DI have suspicions which they feel unable to voice to their parents. One mother whose children are now adult continues to live with this uncertainty:

> Well, I mean, I'm not saying that the children might not have inklings; I mean, who's to say? I don't think perhaps they'd broach the subject with us. But they must put two and two together; eleven years [of marriage before the first baby] is a long time. And my husband has said to my son that we never used any contraceptives, so perhaps they have put two and two together. Who's to say?

How do children react to learning that they were conceived by donor insemination?

Until recently, because of the secrecy that has traditionally surrounded DI, very little has been known about how the children have fared, and even now the information we have is based on the experiences of quite a small number of individuals. Among the families taking part in our interviews we asked the few parents who had told their children they were conceived by DI to describe their children's reactions to this news. The children of these couples were still too young to fully understand what donor insemination meant but they had not been upset. One mother said:

> He wasn't terribly impressed really. He was being awkward when he was asking questions which weren't being directly answered. That was niggling at him more.

We have also made direct contact with a small number of young adults who were aware of their DI origins and who were willing to explore and discuss at length their reactions to learning about this. When they were eventually told, all these young adults had accepted their DI status equably and none of them had found it a particularly traumatic experience. One young man said: 'It even surprised me that it didn't upset me particularly.' Another young woman was quite excited at the thought that she had been conceived by DI and that this made her a kind of pioneer: 'I was sort of *pleased* in a way—being one of the first people to be born in this way by DI.' These young people had certainly been surprised when they were told, but some of that surprise was because their parents had felt the need to keep the matter such a close secret for so many years. None of them regretted the fact that their parents had had them by DI. They were enjoying life and happy to be alive and realised that they owed their existence to DI. They were also pleased to feel that their parents had wanted a child so badly, and that they were the child who had fulfilled their parents' wishes. One said:

> . . . the realisation that I'd been brought into the world, you know, they actually went to *tremendous* lengths because they wanted to have a baby. And I suddenly felt that they must love me a tremendous amount, that I was very important to them.

In the cases where the father was still alive and in contact with the child, the fear that the father/child relationship would be damaged proved to be unfounded. Indeed, the relationship in some cases had been strengthened as the son or daughter came to realise the anguish which the father must at times have experienced.

> To me he's my father. And realising the trauma they must have been through, having this huge, great secret and trying to keep it from me—you know I have tremendous respect for them.

The young people were not overly curious about the identity of the anonymous donor who had donated his semen and they did not appear to spend time worrying about who he was. Nor did they seem to have any lack of self-identity or a sense of not being sure who they were. That side of things had not bothered them at all. They had identified with the father who had brought them up and without exception considered him to be their father. This is similar to the experience of adopted children who discover the identity of their biological parents when they are older. Some of these young adults had suspected that something was different in their relationship with their parents; two had queried their eye colour, another had discussed his doubts about his paternity with an adopted sister, and another had queried his blood group. But this last young man also said:

> It was just a general thing—it was as if I'd always known there was something wrong, I'd always known there was something amiss and suddenly, being told that, it was as if a huge great weight had been lifted off my shoulders.

From the experience of this small number of young adults it would seem that many of the fears expressed by parents about their children are likely to be unfounded. Parents have found it possible to explain DI origins to their children. This knowledge has not damaged the personality of the child nor does it appear to have disrupted close family relationships. What is more, these young people appear to be pleased that they have, at last, been told.

At what age is it best to tell a child that he or she was conceived by donor insemination?

The young people we have referred to were all told when they were young adults, normally in their late teens or early twenties. However, most people are agreed that children should normally be told about their biological origins at a much younger age. There is no one specific age when it is best to give this information. Nor is it likely a child (of any age) could be told—and take in and understand—all the relevant facts at one time. It is much more a matter of a child gradually beginning to absorb and learn the relevant knowledge over a considerable period of time, and almost without knowing this is happening. With babies this is how all learning takes place and the earlier one begins to tell a child, the better. The aim is to impart the information so that when adult, the person can say 'I wasn't told; I just always knew.'

When it comes to actually formulating the words which tell the child about his or her donor conception parents can find it very difficult. Some parents have found it is easier to start doing this while the child is still a baby. At this time parents are saying all sorts of intimate things to their baby which the baby does not understand. At this very early stage parents can begin to talk to their baby about their longing and their struggle to have a baby of their own. As these words are repeated the child will later on come to understand what they mean, but by then the parent will have become more used to saying them. In this way the 'story' of the child's life can evolve and enlarge as the child grows and becomes more aware.

With time it is inevitable that the child will begin to ask questions about a wide range of subjects. These questions should be answered truthfully as they crop up in the natural run of family life; more complex questions will come as the child gets older. Each question should be answered truthfully, and at a level of simplicity appropriate to the age of the child. As more questions are asked and answered, a gradual understanding of sexuality in general and about DI will then develop. In this way the child will come to a full understanding of DI without the need for the parents to identify a specific time when the child is told.

How can parents best explain to their child that he or she was conceived by donor insemination?

Information about DI is best given gradually along with other information about sexual matters, and given in a simple way appropriate to the age of the child. As well as the facts of reproduction the child would also have to learn about the possibility of seeking help to achieve a baby when the normal reproductive processes are ineffective. A child would probably have to be rather older in order to fully understand this. Children do not ask all their questions at once, and it is a mistake to give more information than they ask for. To do so will probably only serve to confuse them and to reduce the likelihood of the child understanding the answer to his/her own question. Children may also need to ask the same question several times before they achieve a proper understanding of the answers given.

Parents of adopted children are encouraged to tell their children of their adoption while they are still very young by means of stories, and by emphasising the fact that the adopted child was *chosen* by their adoptive parents. One of the older mothers who shared her experiences with us has two children, an elder son born following DI treatment and a younger, adopted daughter. They are both now grown up and married with children of their own. She had told both these children of their biological origins. She explained how her adopted daughter had always had a favourite bedtime story. In this story her mother and her brother went to a big house where there were lots of babies. These babies were all lying fast asleep in cots in the nursery. Her mother and brother had gone to the big house to choose a baby. They had wanted to take all the babies, but they crept by the cots, one by one, until they came to their *special* baby. Then they gently picked her up out of her cot, carefully wrapped her in a shawl and took her home. This story had been repeated many times. Later, when this daughter was told by her mother that she was adopted, her mother reminded her of the favourite bedtime story and explained how she had been telling her of her adoption all along.

One of the younger couples with whom we have maintained contact are also telling their small daughter about her DI origins most skillfully. When their daughter was very small and without waiting for any questions to be asked, these young parents devised a simple story about their desire for a baby and efforts to conceive. This became their daughter's favourite bedtime story. The child eventually knew 'her' story by heart even though she did not, at first, completely understand it. Her cousins also know this story and some of them have personal stories of their own too which the children share. (One had to be nursed in an incubator because she was so tiny when she was born.) An acquaintance has had a baby following IVF treatment so, as the child's mother said: 'She knows other people do have other babies by other means.' The parents have gradually added more detail to her story and eventually included the need for a donor. By this time (their daughter was now aged 8 years) they thought their daughter had understood about DI, but as a result of a remark she made a few days later it became clear that her understanding was still incomplete. This experience tends to confirm current knowledge about how children learn; repeated explanations are needed and concepts are gradually understood. Indeed, it is this slow and gradual movement towards understanding which spares the child the sudden shock of knowledge about DI and allows the child to grow up feeling that he or she 'has always known'.

When adopted children learn that they are adopted the most hurtful part of this knowledge is that they were relinquished by their biological mother, however good her reasons for giving up her child may have been. The fact that the child was *chosen* by its adoptive parents is deliberately stressed in an attempt to compensate for this feeling of being rejected by the biological mother. In this respect it is much easier to tell a child conceived by DI about its biological origins. A child conceived by DI does not have to cope with any experience of rejection. A DI child is above all else a *wanted* child, a child who was longed for and earnestly desired, and whose birth followed a great deal of planning and resulted in great rejoicing.

Adoptive parents are also advised about the importance of referring to their child's biological parents in a positive and approving way. This helps the child to develop positive feelings about him/herself. It is helpful for the child to know something about the biological parents such as their occupation and their interests and skills; most adopted children are more interested in these broad social details than in the actual identity of their biological parents. In the same way it is important for children who know they were conceived by DI that the donor is referred to in a positive way. This is why it is important for couples having DI treatment to ask the treatment centre for some information about the donor to share with their child at an appropriate time.

A group of parents whose own children were conceived by DI have recently published an excellent children's picture story book called 'My Story' which explains DI in a way in which a young child can understand. They felt there was a need for such a book and so set about producing one themselves. The book is highly recommended; details of where to obtain it can be found in the list of useful publications at the back of this book. In addition, a support group for parents who have decided to tell their child of his/her DI origins or who are trying to make up their minds about this, has recently been set up. An address from where details can be obtained is also given at the back of this book.

We offer the following story as one possible way in which parents could begin to explain to young children about their biological origins. This idea grew out of a remark made by one of the husbands with whom we talked, who referred to the donor's semen being 'lent' to him and his wife to produce the baby they both wanted.

> Daddy was very sad because he didn't have enough seed to make a baby. Mummy was very sad too. They were both sad because it meant they couldn't have a baby. And they wanted a baby very very much. Then a *very* kind man, who had enough seed, said he would

> give some of his seed to Daddy. Because he knew how much Daddy and Mummy wanted their very own baby. We don't know who this man was—just that he was good and kind—and he sent his seed to the hospital so that Daddy and Mummy could have a baby. A doctor put the seed, which the kind man had sent, into Mummy, and so a baby began to grow in her tummy. And Daddy and Mummy were very, very happy because they were going to have their very own baby.

If any parent has a story or script for telling their child which they have successfully used, why not share it with other parents who are, or will be, in a similar position? The support group (address at the back of this book) or the authors of this book would be pleased to help make such scripts available to others.

Useful Addresses

British Agencies for Adoption and Fostering
11 Southwark Street
London SE1 1RQ
(Telephone: 071-407 8800)

'Child'
PO Box 154
Hounslow
Middlesex TW5 0EZ
(Telephone: 081-893 7110)
or
Suite 219
Caledonian House
98 The Centre
Seltham
Middlesex TW13 4BH
(Telephone: 081-844 2468)

Family Planning Association (National Office)
27-35 Mortimer Street
London W1N 7RJ
(Telephone: 071-636 7866)

Human Fertilisation and Embryology Authority
Paxton House
30 Artillery Lane
London E1 7LS
(Telephone: 071-377 5077)

'Issue' (National Fertility Association)
St. George's Rectory
Tower Street
Birmingham B19 3UY
(Telephone: 021-359 4887)

Parent Support Group:
DI Network
PO Box 265
Sheffield
S3 7YX

University of Exeter Press
Reed Hall
Streatham Drive
Exeter EX4 4QR
(For information on how to obtain further copies of this book)

Useful Books

The Infertility Handbook by Sarah J. Biggs.
Available from: Fertility Services Management, The New House, Far End, Sheepscombe, Stroud, Gloucestershire GL6 7RL. 1989 (ISBN 0-9514205-0-X)

Infertility: Modern Treatments and the Issues They Raise by Maggie Jones. Published by Piatkus, London. 1991 (ISBN 0-7499-1031-3)
Available from bookshops.

My Story
Available from: Infertility Research Trust, University Department of Obstetrics and Gynaecology, Jessop Hospital for Women, Sheffield S3 7RE.

Index

Copies of this book can be obtained through booksellers or in case of difficulty by contacting University of Exeter Press at Reed Hall, Streatham Drive, Exeter EX4 4QR